Jessica H

the

pursuit

of

motherhood

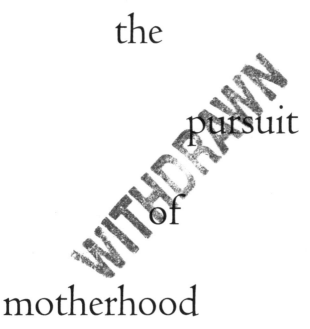

Matador
9 Priory Business Park,
Wistow Road, Kibworth Beauchamp,
Leicestershire. LE8 0RX
Tel: (+44) 116 279 2299
Fax: (+44) 116 279 2277
Email: books@troubador.co.uk
Web: www.troubador.co.uk/matador

ISBN 9781783061877

British Library Cataloguing in Publication Data.
A catalogue record for this book is available from the British Library.

Typeset by Troubador Publishing Ltd, Leicester, UK

Matador is an imprint of Troubador Publishing Ltd

For all the women who know how it feels

Contents

Prologue   1

Smiling Faces   4

Made in 1970   14

Only Human   17

Peter and Me   33

Chemical Attraction   35

Top Girls   49

The Curious Incident of the Spring Roll
    in the Night-Time   52

The 100m Hurdle Race   62

Dreaming Spires   66

Out Damned Spot   75

What a Difference a Day Makes   77

Socks and Stairs   91

Shit Happens   93

The Fool   105

Mini-Molly   109

Jerusalem   118

Anger Management   122

The Stonemasons Arms 129

The Point 133

It's Different for Boys 141

Hope You're Happy Too 144

Shift Happens 146

Price Pritchett 156

Inadequate 159

Thoughts on Therapy 169

Mr T 171

Doritos (Family Size) 181

Zebras and Leopards 188

Show Me the Evidence 196

The Secret Cycle 201

Money 207

Natural Selection 211

The Other Options 218

601 Days 221

Blessings 229

Epilogue 231

Acknowledgements 235

PROLOGUE

It's a Sunday in September. It should be autumn but feels like summer. As I put my make-up on in the car mirror, I start to count the number of babies that our friends and family have had since we began trying to conceive.

'Vicky: two. Beth: two. Joanne: two. Sarah Jane: two. Jo: two. Antonia: two. Harriet: one. Mel: one. Caroline: three!' My voice crescendos on the number three.

Peter glances over at me.

'Are you going to be OK?' he asks.

'That's seventeen babies. One more isn't going to make it any harder,' I say, leaning into the mirror to take advantage of a few moments at a red light to apply my eyeliner.

We're on our way to a family lunch. My cousin, who now lives in Peru, has just come over to the UK with her husband and their new baby – number eighteen. We're late, as usual. I've actually been up since 4 a.m. finishing a report for work but Peter couldn't drag me away from the computer. I flip up the car mirror, reach for my mobile phone and text:

Sorry. Running Late. Don't put our dinner in the dog :)

When we arrive pre-lunch rituals are already in full swing. Adults chatting; children playing; delicious smells emanating from the oven. Someone thrusts a glass of Prosecco into my hand. I take a large gulp. My cousin and her Peruvian husband, Guillermo, look so relaxed and happy, with eyes for no one but each other and their beautiful baby.

'So…' Guillermo says, pulling himself away from his new daughter. 'How's work?'

The first question everyone asks me.

'Busy,' I say. 'Good busy, though. I've just raised a lot of money to build an extension to the theatre.'

'Wow. That sounds exciting.'

'Yes, it is, I guess.'

I can tell I sound distracted. With my other ear I am straining to hear a conversation that has just started across the kitchen and I've never been good at doing two things at the same time. They are talking about the wife of another cousin of mine who got married just a few months ago.

I overhear someone saying: 'Well, if you do the maths, she must have conceived on the actual day of the wedding, or thereabouts.'

'Yes,' someone else says. 'And she looks fabulous with a bit of weight on her.'

I look down into my half-drunk glass of Prosecco as my stomach lurches with an all-too-familiar feeling. Time to add another name to the list of all the women for whom getting pregnant seems to be as easy as the simple steps in the book my mother bought me when I was a little girl: *How Mummy and Daddy Make a Baby*.

All the women, that is, except me.

SMILING FACES

'Bottle of Chardonnay?' Vicky says, throwing her things down on the chair and taking her purse out of her bag.

Tara and I both murmur our approval.

'And get some crisps,' I call after her. 'I can't drink without a canapé.'

'What flavour?' she calls back. 'I know you're particular about these things.'

'Plain,' I say decisively. 'You *can* only have plain crisps with white wine.'

'You mean *you* can only have plain crisps with white wine,' Tara says, smiling at me.

I'm on an evening out with a bunch of old school friends. The fact that Tara's here makes it extra special. She emigrated to Australia a few years ago and rarely comes back to London. For old times' sake, we've chosen to meet up at the Railway Tavern, although it's not actually called that any more. A few years ago, around about the time we were all turning thirty, it became a gastropub and was renamed the Garden Gate, which sounds much more like the sort of place you'd go to have fishcakes. But for us it will always be just 'the Railway', venue for my eighteenth birthday party (messy), many a hard-fought pool tournament (for the record I've never been good at pool, so I'm glad those days are over), and toilet tears (so many toilet tears).

'Isn't it funny how much things have changed?' Tara says while Vicky is at the bar. 'In the old days it would have been a bottle of Lambrusco and a packet of ten Silk Cut.'

'Do you think they still make Lambrusco?'

'They should do. It was the cure for everything.'

'It was,' I laugh.

'And do you remember how we always said that I would be the first to have a baby because you'd be too busy focusing on your career.'

'And my penthouse apartment.'

'Yes. Sorry. And your penthouse apartment.'

'Not sure what happened to the penthouse…'

'London property prices.'

'That and choosing a career in the arts. Anyway, Ta, I've not had a baby yet. We're still working on it.'

'You will soon though,'

'And so will you.'

'Gotta meet the right person first. There's just the small problem of supply and demand.'

'What do you mean?'

'I mean there's too much demand and not enough supply.'

'Yeah, why are there so many more attractive, intelligent, successful single women in their thirties than there are men?'

'I don't know, but feminism has a lot to answer for.'

Vicky comes back from the bar as another of our school friends, Beth, arrives.

'Glass of white OK?' Vicky asks her.

'Perfect,' Beth replies.

Vicky pours four large glasses.

'So Vic, I take it there's no need for me to start knitting yet,' Tara says, pointing at her wine glass.

Vicky got married last summer and, like me, she is also trying for her first baby.

'No news yet,' she says. 'We've been at it like rabbits for over six months though.'

'Snap!' I say.

'I've got some news,' Beth interrupts suddenly.

'Yes?' We all turn to her.

'Thomas and I have decided to start trying.'

Beth and Thomas got together last year so you could say that this is relatively fast work. But I won't.

'That's great,' Vicky says. 'We can all be yummy mummies together.'

'Yummy mummies and their maiden aunt,' Tara jokes.

I kick her under the table.

'So here's some advice,' Vicky says to Beth. 'Get

yourself down to the chemist tomorrow and buy yourself an ovulation predictor kit.'

'A what?' Beth asks.

'It basically tells you the two days each month you are most likely to conceive,' I explain. 'Contrary to what Mrs Smith told us in biology, it doesn't just happen as soon as you stop using contraception.'

'Do you remember those classes?' Tara says. 'I still feel sorry for her. She was so much more comfortable talking about photosynthesis.'

We all laugh and then raise our glasses to old friends and Mrs Smith's biology lessons.

'I wish I'd known about the ovulation thingy earlier,' Vicky continues. 'I feel like we wasted the first few months.'

'Relax, Vic,' I say. 'I've read loads of stuff that says it's completely normal for it to take up to a year to get pregnant.'

'I've read that too,' says Beth. 'Especially if you've been on the pill.'

'We all need to stop worrying…' I say sagely as I lick the crisp salt off my fingers and take another sip of wine. 'And just keep on having lots of fun trying.'

Yeah. Right.

Like many women of my generation, I didn't even think about having a baby until I was in my thirties. Anytime before that would have been – for want of a better word – *uncool*. I went to an all-girls comprehensive which was renowned for turning out independent, career-driven young women. Getting married and having a family was something you assumed you'd do when you were older. Much older. I didn't break the mould.

When the school careers adviser asked me what I wanted to do when I grew up, I said that I wanted either to run a theatre or become an expedition leader and travel the world. He didn't bat an eyelid. Motherhood didn't figure in any of my dreams when I was eighteen and the thought of being a young mother was not only an embarrassment but anathema. Along with most of my friends, I spent my twenties pursuing my career. By my early thirties, I was running one of London's leading theatres. It would have made my careers adviser proud.

I had just turned thirty-four when Peter and I first started trying for a baby. (If you could wind back and ask my eighteen-year-old self what the perfect age was, I'd probably have said this was it.) We had been together nearly four years and the topic had been under discussion for a while. Then, one Christmas Day, just as we were sitting down to dinner with my family, Peter looked at me across the table and mouthed: 'Let's do it!' It was one of those movie moments when, for a few seconds, our eyes locked and it was as if we were the only two people in the world.

Soon after we finished Christmas pudding and coffee, we made our excuses to leave. Compelled by our silent exchange across the dinner table, we were desperate to see how it felt to be alone with such a momentous decision. It felt good. In fact, it felt good for weeks, as we had a lot of fun having sex for the purpose that it was originally intended. We even decided to have a ritual throwing-away of all the contraception in the bathroom cupboard – condoms, pills, the cap I never got on with and which hardly left its box. It was a good reason for opening a bottle of bubbly.

'It's kind of a like a pre-wetting of the baby's head,' Peter said.

I laughed. 'Does that mean you've stashed away a couple of boxes of condoms so we can have another pre-wetting tomorrow?'

One month of unadulterated love-making later, it was a bit of surprise when my period arrived and I hadn't got pregnant. Ditto the following month. But then, it must be one of the most successful fallacies of 1980s sex education that Man + Woman + Unprotected Sex = Pregnancy. It's actually quite a complicated process.

Most months most women release one egg from

their ovaries (there are two of them – ovaries that is – one on the left and one on the right). Both are filled with tiny follicles containing eggs, and from the first day of your period it takes approximately two weeks for them to mature. At this point the largest follicle releases an egg, which heads off down one of your two fallopian tubes. Here, it relies on meeting an active and able sperm, which then has to bury itself into the egg in order to fertilise it. As sperm only survive for a few days, there's just a small window of opportunity for everything to be in the right place at the right time for conception to occur. It's kind of a miracle that so many people manage it.

Now of course this is how it's meant to happen, and you do hear all sorts of stories about women getting pregnant at unusual times. But for most women, most of the time, conception only occurs in the middle of their monthly cycle. If we'd known that when we were teenagers, it might have saved a lot of distraught late-night telephone calls to friends.

A few months in and we start to focus our efforts around the right time. With this a whole new phase begins. *Sex To Order*. It doesn't matter how tired we are or how much we're in the mood: come the middle of the month, I demand we have sex. It brings a whole new meaning to the word 'dominatrix'. Fun at first. But only at first.

A few months after that, still with no results, we

progress to the ovulation predictor kit, a clever little thing that, like Beth, I didn't even know existed until we started trying for a baby. The kit is designed to detect the onset of ovulation – the moment when your egg leaves your ovaries – from a surge in the hormone known as LH (the luteinising hormone), which can be measured in your urine. To maximise your chance of conceiving, you should have sex within forty-eight hours of the surge taking place. There are several types of kit available. I like the one that shows a smiling face when it detects the LH increase. Partly because it's the easiest one to read, and partly because it's such a lovely symbol of hope that everything is working properly and the time is right.

I soon discover, however, that although the ovulation predictor kit might improve the accuracy of our mid-cycle sex, it also brings with it a further sense of imperative. The moment I see that smiling face, we start to have fractious conversations about when and where we're going to make it work. We already have busy lives and it becomes yet another urgent meeting that we have to fit into our diaries. One morning I get the smiling face when Peter's staying out of town for a couple of nights, working. I ring him with a plan.

'You're going to have to drive back late tomorrow night otherwise we'll miss another month,' I say. 'We'll already be thirty-six hours in, but maybe we can do it a couple of times during the night to make up for it.'

'Don't you think quality is better than quantity?'

'No. I think we need to get as many of the bloody buggers up there as possible.'

'You're so romantic,' he says.

'Romance is overrated. This is business.'

The following night the phone rings. It's Peter. He sounds tired.

'Would you mind if I set off really early tomorrow morning and we can do it before you go to work?' he asks. 'We'll still be in time, won't we?'

'It's cutting it fine. But OK, just as long as you're here by seven. I need to leave by eight.'

At 6 a.m. I am awake and waiting. When I ring Peter to check on his progress, I discover he's overslept and is still in his hotel room. Another month lost. Another fractious conversation. But even when the timings work out, getting your kecks off and getting on with it is hardly the best way of making love or conceiving a child.

The one consolation in all of this is that in the early days of us trying to conceive, I'm not on my own. Lots of my girlfriends are going through exactly the same thing. But gradually their fun delivers results, whereas Peter and I have month after month after month of smiling faces and nothing whatsover to smile about.

The Infertility Diaries Part I

I opened the newspaper today and saw the headline 'GENERATION X PUTS WORK BEFORE KIDS'. The first sentence read: 'They were supposed to have it all but nearly half the university-educated women in Generation X – born between 1965 and 1978 – have no children.'

I was born in 1970. I have a career. I don't have children. I guess on the face of it the statisticians would include me in their hypothesis.

In the article they describe these women (me!) as 'child-free' rather than 'childless'. It's a subtle distinction but the implication is that we have actively chosen work over having a family.

I haven't.

My own theory – not statistically proven, of course – is that women of my generation who don't have children actually fall into one of three categories:

1. *Women who have a career and don't want children;*
2. *Women who have a career and do want children but can't find the right partner;*
3. *Women who have a career, do want children, do have a partner but can't get pregnant.*

As for the women who do have children, well, they've either had to sacrifice their career, or I suppose they must have it all. (And frankly, if there is any woman out there who has achieved that Generation X dream, then I don't think I want to know as it will only make me feel like a failure.)

I am Category Three. I have a career and a partner but I can't get pregnant. I'm pretty sure that if I had got pregnant when we first started trying, my career would have stalled. But that would be another story…

MADE IN 1970

Here are some other things it might be useful to know about me:

I was born and brought up in London – north not south, a distinction that is very important to the indigenous community of the capital.

I essentially grew up as an only child. I've got one half-sister – from my mum's first marriage – but she's much older than me, and left home to live with her boyfriend when I was only four.

When I was six, my teacher announced that the person in the class with the largest family could take home the Halloween pumpkin. I took her aside at the end of the day and told her there were nine of us – my mum, my dad, three sisters, three brothers and me.

A few weeks later, I overheard my teacher saying

to my mum: 'I do feel for you. It must be a lot of work with all your children.'

'Not really,' my mum said brightly. 'I only have the two.'

I kept my head down. The way I figured it, the basis for awarding the pumpkin was unfair anyway. I always wanted a big family. It wasn't my fault that my mum and dad didn't have one.

I wasn't the '-est' anything at school. The prettiest, the cleverest, the funniest, the naughtiest (believe me, that pumpkin lie was nothing in an inner-London state school). I've never played the lottery because I know I'm not the luckiest. I strongly believe it's the '-ests' that define us. If you ask any of my friends they'd probably say I work the hardest of most people they know.

I have been an obsessive list-maker all my life. I have lists of all the books I've read; all the countries I've been to; all the things I want to do before I die. If our house caught fire, my little library of list-books would be the first thing I'd grab from the burning building.

My guilty pleasures include eating out at nice restaurants, staying in posh hotels, and buying new season when I'm supposed to be shopping in the sales. I have expensive tastes and modest means. Any month in which my income exceeds my expenditure is an occasion for celebration – which often means that next month I'm back in the red.

I love food, but please don't give me carrots and tomatoes in the same dish. In fact, any combination of red and orange on the same plate is a no-no. I'm also very particular about olives. I only eat even numbers, although I can do five at a push. Apart from that I'm a perfect dinner party guest. I eat everything. Oh, except caviar. It's a texture thing; I don't like the way it pops in your mouth.

Like everyone, I have my weaknesses and weirdness. When infertility happens you can't help wondering whether these have anything to do with it.

The Infertility Diaries Part II

One of the things you notice when you start trying hard to have a baby is that the world is full of pregnant women. The strange thing is, I never noticed them before. But now they're everywhere. They're walking towards me on every street; they're all over the television, looking glamorous; and they're on the Tube with their 'Baby on Board' badges, just in case I didn't notice them in the crush.

ONLY HUMAN

Around a year after we begin trying for a baby it becomes clear that not a lot is happening. CORRECTION: nothing is happening.

I find myself staying late at work, googling things like: 'Why can't I get pregnant?' Incidentally, this is the fifth most commonly asked question on the Internet with the suffix 'Why can't I...' The most popular being 'Why can't I own a Canadian?' Hmmm...

One evening I decide to broach the subject with Peter.

'Shall we sit at the table for supper tonight?' I suggest.

He looks at me, immediately suspicious.

'What's wrong with the sofa suddenly?' he asks.

'There's something I want to talk to you about...'

'That sounds ominous.'

'It's just that I've been doing some thinking...'

'What have I told you about that?' he says. 'Thinking is never a good idea – especially where you're concerned.'

He laughs at his own joke and starts to lay the cutlery out on the table whilst I dish up. We sit down ceremoniously.

'So how was your day?' I ask.

'Now I'm *really* worried. What *is* it you want to talk about?'

'It's nothing much. I've just been wondering whether we should go and see a fertility doctor. It's been over a year and nothing's happened.'

'It's probably me,' he says immediately.

It's the first time I've even thought about one of us being to blame. I suddenly realise that this must be hard for him too.

'Why do you think that?'

'Well, you're always telling me that I'm not healthy enough…'

'Yes, that's true, but it can't be the only reason. Anyway, I've been doing some research –'

'You've obviously been thinking about this a lot.'

'I have had a few chats with Mr Google.'

He smiles.

'So what do you and Mr Google think we should do?'

'We could go on the NHS. But it might take a lot of time so maybe we should pay.'

'Won't it be expensive?'

'An initial appointment is about a hundred quid. It should also be easier to organise appointments around work.'

'If that's what you want.'

'It's not exactly what I want… but I do want a baby.'

'I want us to have one too,' he says gently. And then: '*Now* can we go and sit on the sofa?'

I am embarrassed to admit that my initial research into the world of fertility clinics is pretty rudimentary. In fact, the main reason behind my choice of clinic is that it's based at the central London hospital where I was born. I am totally oblivious to league tables. I do a basic Internet search and choose familiarity over live birth rates. I don't even know what live birth rates are.

I ring the clinic. They take both NHS and private patients and because I'm prepared to pay they offer us an appointment in a few weeks' time.

Whilst it feels good to be doing something proactive about the situation, as the day of our appointment edges closer I feel myself becoming increasingly apprehensive, as a whole new layer of anxiety – *my fear of human fallibility* – starts to spread over the base-coat of disappointment that I am already dealing with. The day before our appointment I snap at Peter because I can't find the measuring jug he's put away in the wrong cupboard. He looks at me.

'What is going on with you at the moment?' he asks.

'Nothing. Why?'

'You've just got cross with me about a measuring jug.'

'So?'

'Misplacing it is hardly a heinous crime.'

'Sorry,' I concede. 'I think I'm a bit nervous about tomorrow.'

'Why? I thought you'd be excited.'

'I am. But I can't stop thinking that we shouldn't have to do this to make a baby. It seems unnatural.'

'Lots of couples have problems conceiving.'

'I know, but it feels like cheating.'

'Sometimes that's the only way to win.'

'I also keep worrying that they're going to make a mistake. That I'll end up having someone else's baby and we won't even know.'

'Aren't you rushing ahead a bit? We haven't even had our first appointment yet.'

I take a bottle of milk out of the fridge and start to pour it into the missing – now found – measuring jug. I know he's right. As usual I'm hurtling headlong to all the worst conclusions. It's the pessimist in me.

I'm not sure what I expected a fertility clinic to feel like before I went to one. It wasn't something I had given a lot of thought. But if I had thought about it, I don't think I would have expected it to feel like this. We walk through the main doors of the hospital – which look just like your average hospital doors. We follow a long corridor – which looks just like your average hospital corridor. Then up two flights of stairs and through another nondescript door before emerging into a room with panelled wooden walls, heavy oak furniture and wingback chairs. It looks more like the setting of a Dickens' novel than a twenty-first-century NHS hospital. It's surreal. It definitely doesn't feel like the sort of place you go to create a baby.

The next shock is the other people. The waiting room is full of them. Men and women, all of whom look completely normal and fertile but clearly aren't. I can tell from the thickness of their patient files that some are at the beginning of their infertility journey and some have been travelling for years. But none of them look or speak to one another. We all sit in silence, side-by-side, wishing we didn't have to be there and secretly wondering why everyone else is.

Eventually Peter and I are called through to see the doctor, who, sitting on the other side of a large desk, leans over to shake our hands and introduce himself. He asks the obvious questions. How old are we? How long have we been trying to conceive? Is there anything in our medical history that we think could have affected our fertility? Sadly none of the answers to these questions can solve anything immediately. The first stage of the infertility process is tests. These end up taking about a month to complete. They involve checking the quantity and quality of Peter's sperm, and finding out whether I am producing eggs and if they have a clear passage from my ovaries, through my fallopian tubes, and into my uterus.

At the end of this, our tests prove conclusive in their inconclusiveness and we are diagnosed with what is described as 'unexplained infertility'. Although the doctor tells us that, technically, this means there is no reason we can't get pregnant, I quickly realise that it actually means he has no idea why we're not. This makes it one of the worst forms of infertility, as it's so much easier to 'fix' something when you know what the problem is. IVF, for example, was specifically invented for women who had blocked fallopian tubes. Through the process of IVF their eggs were surgically removed, fertilised outside the body and then put back into the uterus, bypassing their fallopian tubes altogether. Hey presto, they'd found the solution to the problem. But when you don't know what the problem is, it can be difficult, maybe impossible, to find the solution.

It turns out that for most couples diagnosed with unexplained infertility the first treatment prescribed is a process call intrauterine insemination (IUI for short). It's kind of like IVF-lite. The clinic simply monitors you until you ovulate and then at the optimum moment inserts your partner's sperm – which has been pre-produced and filtered in the laboratory – directly into your uterus using a syringe. The aim of this is simply to make sure that everything is in the right place at the right time to do things naturally.

I listen carefully whilst our doctor explains the process to us.

'So,' he says, coming to a close. 'IUI is a relatively cost-effective and straightforward process that I suggest you try two or three times before you consider progressing to IVF.'

'OK,' says Peter. 'That sounds doable. When do we start?'

'On your next cycle, if you like.' The doctor turns to me. 'Do you know when your period is due, Jessica?'

'Erm…before we look at dates, there's just something I need to ask you.'

I look at him. And then at Peter, who already knows what I'm going to say.

'Yes?' the doctor says.

'I know this might be irrational,' I say tentatively, 'but would it be possible for us to sit with the sperm while it's being prepared in the laboratory?'

'Why would you want to do that?' he asks with surprise.

'I know, it sounds stupid…but I have this horrible fear of Peter's sperm being mixed up with someone else's. It would really help me if we could be with it at all times.'

He looks at me askance. 'I understand your concerns, Ms Hepburn,' he says. 'You've read about the case in Leeds. You don't want to risk the possibility of having a *black* baby.'

He lingers on the word 'black'.

I stare at him aghast. I can hardly believe what he has just said. The special thing about deciding to have a baby with someone you love is that you are creating a new human being together. I want to experience what it feels like for people to look at our child and say that it's got my eyes and Peter's nose (actually that wouldn't be such a good combination, but you know what I mean).

'That's not it at all…' I stammer. 'I don't want anyone else's baby. Whatever the colour. I want *Peter's* baby.'

'I can assure you, Ms Hepburn, our laboratory procedures are very rigorous,' he continues. 'Every action is witnessed by two people, making the possibility of a mix-up extremely unlikely. I'm afraid we can't allow you into the lab because we have to protect the confidentiality of other patients.'

He pauses and looks at me. I think he can tell how tense and afraid I am.

'Look,' he says more gently. 'I'll have a word with the senior embryologist. I can't promise anything but I'll see what I can do.'

As soon as I get home, I turn on the computer and google: *Fertility Treatment Mix-up, Leeds*. It appears the case involved a black baby that was born to two white parents. A further trawl of the Internet throws up dozens of other fertility treatment mix-ups. Although it is ironic that human endeavour and achievement might be the only thing that makes it possible for us to have a baby, it just confirms and deepens my paranoia about the process. People make mistakes. It doesn't matter how good they are at their job; they're only human.

Peter comes into the room and I quickly close my laptop.

'What are you doing?' he asks.

'Nothing.'

'Google is a very dangerous thing, you know.' He looks at me for a long second. 'We don't have to go through with this if you don't want to.'

'Of course I want to go through with it. I just need to be sure that they're going to put your sperm inside me and not someone else's.'

'You're going have to trust them.'

'But this is such a horrible thing to have to go through. You'd think they'd want to do everything they can to make patients feel as relaxed as possible.'

'You've got to respect that they have a way of doing things. They can't change it just for you.'

'We're paying. Surely that counts for something.'

'I'm not sure it does. Judging by the number of the people in the waiting room this is clearly a sellers' market.'

'But this isn't a straightforward business transaction. I'm not just buying a can of Coke.'

'The problem is you don't like it when you're not in control.'

'The problem is I never knew that having a baby was something that I wouldn't have any control over.'

The next day I get a call from the senior embryologist at the clinic. It's clear that he's not particularly happy about my request to witness our treatment either. No one likes to feel mistrusted and procedures are power, so I do understand. However, after a long conversation he reluctantly agrees that I can sit outside the lab and watch the sperm preparation through a hatch. With this confirmed, our introduction to IUI begins. I am monitored during the first part of my monthly cycle to ensure everything is progressing as planned. Then, approximately fourteen days in, we are told to report for duty the following morning.

When we arrive at the clinic, the receptionist suggests I take a seat in the waiting room whilst Peter goes downstairs to produce his 'sample'. This was something we had also discussed with the doctor. In an attempt to make the process as close to the real thing as possible, we had asked whether I could be there when Peter produces his sperm sample. For me, it's tantamount to being at our child's conception. The doctor had looked at me quizzically again, but said that he was sure it could be arranged. It was, apparently, an *unusual* but not an *unheard-of* request.

The receptionist gives us the same quizzical expression. (Note to fertility receptionists everywhere: just a little more empathy wouldn't go amiss in recognition of the fact that men masturbating in a room on their own is not the way most of us imagined we would make a baby).

She picks up the phone and calls a colleague: 'Can you please take a gentleman downstairs to produce a sample. Oh, and…' she pauses as if for effect, 'Ms Hepburn wants to come too.'

Please! Tell everyone, why don't you?! So much for that all-important patient confidentiality.

A nurse comes through and takes us to what is known as the 'producing room', although really it can hardly pass as a room at all. It is more like a cupboard. There is a table on one side piled high with boxes of surgical gloves. A bucket and mop in the corner. And a green plastic chair with a couple of well-leafed top-shelf magazines lying underneath. Perhaps it's assumed that men can masturbate anytime anyplace. Perhaps some of them can. Even so, a little bit of extra thought could make the whole experience immeasurably more palatable. A bit of space. A bed, perhaps. Some soft lighting. Maybe an iPod with a selection of music. Especially for couples like us – *unusual* but not *unheard-of* (and maybe not that unusual if couples were routinely given the choice) – who want to be together when their sperm sample is produced so we can say to our child in years to come, 'I was there.'

We look around in incredulous horror.

'Is this it?' I ask her.

'I'm afraid so,' she says. 'Good luck.'

We shut and lock the door.

'How about I lay my coat on the floor?' Peter says.

'OK,' I say. 'Let's give it a go.'

Twenty minutes later and the deed is done. I don't think either of us can get beyond the feeling that lying on Peter's coat in what is essentially a broom-cupboard is not how it ought to be. But we also laugh a lot and feel triumphant at our success.

As we emerge, specimen jar in hand, a nurse intercepts us in the corridor and offers to take it through to the lab. When I explain to her that I'm coming with it she looks uncertain, but a moment later one of the embryologists comes over and confirms that this has been agreed.

Peter goes off to sit in the waiting room whilst I

am kitted out with shoe covers and hair net and taken to a stool by a hatch that opens into the lab. I watch while the embryologist transfers the sperm into a test tube and then puts it into a machine which separates out the best quality ones. This all takes about fifteen minutes to complete. Afterwards she comes over and says that the sample needs to settle for a while before it's ready to go inside me, and that it might be easiest for me to wait outside. She tells me that they need to start working on some other samples (she mentions that old patient confidentiality thing again) and assures me that the sperm won't be moved.

I reluctantly agree and go off to join Peter in the waiting room. Where we wait. And we wait. And we wait. I am acutely aware of time passing but keep thinking that someone will come and get us at any minute.

More than an hour later no one has.

I get up and go over to the receptionist to ask if she can find out how much longer it's going to be.

'What are you in for?' she asks vaguely.

'IUI. We're just waiting to have our sperm put in.'

'OK, I'll check,' she says, and gets up and goes out into the corridor.

After a little while the doors open and she comes back in with a nurse who looks distinctly embarrassed.

'I'm really sorry you've been waiting so long,' the

nurse says, flustered. 'We're just getting things ready for you now.'

She turns and bustles back through the door.

I lean over to Peter. 'They'd forgotten us, hadn't they?'

'Seems that way,' he replies.

A few minutes later the same nurse comes back and calls my name. We are led through to the lobby area just outside the lab where I sat looking through the hatch earlier.

'I'm sorry,' the nurse says. 'All our consultation rooms are busy right now. We're going to have to do the procedure here. Don't worry, though, we'll bring a couple of screens through for privacy. Can you get up on that trolley, please? The doctor will be here in a minute.'

I look at Peter. It is my second look of incredulous horror that day.

'I'm sure it will be fine,' he says quietly. But he doesn't sound so sure.

Then a doctor comes through and introduces himself. It's not one we've met before. He scans my notes then calls out to the embryologist to bring the sperm over. Having waited for ages, everything is now happening very quickly. She emerges with a test tube that I instantly see isn't the same one that I left over an hour ago.

'It's a different test tube,' I blurt out.

The embryologist looks defensive. The doctor looks confused.

'You promised me it wasn't going to move from the one that it was in,' I say anxiously.

'We have to transfer it into a different tube for the insemination,' the embryologist says.

'But why didn't you tell me? Why didn't you let me come and watch? I know you probably think I'm being irrational. Maybe I am. But can't you see this is really difficult for me?'

The embryologist looks defensive again. She moves towards the doctor, who still looks confused. As she does so, I turn to Peter.

'I don't think I can go through with it,' I whisper.

'You can,' he says encouragingly. 'It will be fine.'

'No, I can't.' This time more definite.

'Why don't I ask them for a bit more time?'

'No.' I can feel the tremble in my voice. 'This isn't how it should be. This isn't how I want it to be.'

'I know,' he says.

'Will you tell them for me?' I say with more urgency.

'Are you sure?' he says.

'I'm sure I'm sure.'

So Peter pulls the doctor and embryologist aside to explain while I get dressed. I start to cry. Quietly, but uncontrollably. They look puzzled and mildly concerned, but the doctor soon moves on to his next patient and the embryologist takes the test tube back to the lab.

Looking back, I sometimes wonder what they said when they discussed my case in their weekly team meeting. That's assuming they had a weekly team meeting at which they discussed me. Was I simply dismissed as being an overly neurotic patient? Or did they consider, even for a moment, that I was someone at the beginning of a frightening journey who perhaps needed just a little bit more support? I'm only human, after all.

But I'll never know. I didn't go back. And they never contacted me again.

The Infertility Diaries Part III

When you look at all the people in fertility clinics today, it's extraordinary to remember that less than forty years ago the world's first IVF babies were received with so much fear and loathing. A headline on the front cover of the New York Times *famously heralded the birth of the world's first IVF baby as 'FRANKENSTEIN MYTH BECOMES A REALITY'. Not so much a miracle, then, but a monster. Four million births later, I can't help feeling that the atmosphere of fertility clinics today shows that somewhere, albeit subconsciously,*

that stigma still exists. One of the hardest things about
starting fertility treatment is facing off the enduring opinion
that human beings should never meddle with what nature
decides.

PETER AND ME

Peter and I got together in what I can only describe
as inauspicious circumstances. We worked together
and were both in other relationships when we met.
We always got on well, went out for the occasional
drink to chat about the office, but it was never
anything more than a vaguely flirtatious friendship.
Then one evening, just a few weeks before I was
due to leave the company we both worked for
and move out of town, we ended up in a bar.
Drunk.

There were other people with us at first, but one
by one they peeled off and went home until it was
just us and a kiss that changed everything. As soon
as it happened I grabbed my things, said I had to go,
and ran out of the bar. I stumbled through the
streets angry and ashamed. Peter ran after me,
trying to console me and offering to take me home.
I begged him to leave me alone. He eventually did.

The next thing I could remember was finding myself lying amongst a heap of rubbish bags on the high street. I pulled out my mobile phone and rang my boyfriend, who was away that night on business.

'Where the hell are you?' he said.

'I'm lying in a pile of rubbish,' I said. 'The most terrible thing has just happened.'

'What?'

'I kissed Peter.'

'Peter who?'

'Peter from work.'

'Oh.'

'I feel terrible. I don't know how it happened. I'm drunk.'

'Yes.'

'Very drunk.'

'Yes.'

'What shall I do?'

'Well, right now, you need to get up. You need to walk to the end of the street. And you need to get a taxi to take you home. The rest we'll talk about in the morning.'

He was a lovely guy, my boyfriend, but within a month I'd left him and Peter and I had moved in together. It wasn't an easy decision. It was the hardest, most painful decision I've ever made in my life. But an unexpected kiss unleashed something in both of us. There was nothing we could do but follow it.

CHEMICAL ATTRACTION

I'm not going to make the same mistake again. The next time around I do my research. I get a list of all the clinics in London, order them in terms of their success rates, and start to ring them one by one. The first question I ask is whether they will allow me to witness my treatment. At every call I draw a blank until, finally, someone suggests I contact a small clinic near Regent's Park. They are prepared to consider it, and I make an appointment.

I am already getting accustomed to the oddness of fertility clinics. This one is on the ground floor of a modern apartment building and has a distinctively Scandinavian feel, all blond wood and smooth lines. The doctor who sees us reviews the results of the tests we have already done. He picks up on the fact that one of the tests indicates that Peter's sperm may not be very motile (in other words they don't swim very fast). He says that this might not necessarily be significant but suggests that

Peter performs a sperm survival test as a follow-up.

A few weeks later – test completed – we receive a letter. It says that whilst Peter's sperm count is very good, and the motility reasonable, the survival rate is low. In fact, after twenty-four hours most of the sperm that were still moving were just shaking on the spot. We have to laugh. The thought of Peter's sperm all lined up doing the hokey cokey but not actually getting anywhere. T-y-p-i-c-a-l.

The main problem, the doctor explains at our next appointment, is that it takes twenty-four hours for the sperm to bury into the egg and fertilise it. If Peter's aren't able to survive that long it may be difficult for us to conceive naturally. But, at the same time, he makes a point of emphasising that it doesn't provide a definitive reason as to why I'm not getting pregnant. With millions of sperm in every sample, all you need is for one of them to go the distance, and the probability is that there's going to be at least one that will. Nevertheless, given that we have now been unsuccessfully trying to conceive for nearly two years, his strong suggestion is that we progress directly to IVF and, in our particular case, a treatment called ICSI (intra-cytoplasmic sperm injection). This is essentially just a form of IVF, but instead of letting the egg and sperm fertilise naturally in a Petri dish, an embryologist chops off the sperm's tail and injects the head directly into the egg in order to aid fertilisation. The advantage of this, in our case, is that Peter's sperm won't need to keep kicking for twenty-four hours as there's no swimming work required.

'So?' I say to Peter as we leave the clinic.

'So what?' he replies.

'Do you think we should go through with it?'

'Of course.'

'You make it sound so simple.'

'It is. We want a baby, don't we?'

'But like this?' I say.

'There don't seem to be any other options.'

'I suppose not. But what about the money?'

'We'll find a way.'

'Maybe we should have tried on the NHS first.'

'You'd have even less control if we'd done that. At least this clinic has agreed we can witness everything.'

'Yes, but it's obvious they think we're a bit mad.'

'*We're* a bit mad?'

'OK. *I'm* a bit mad.'

He turns and looks at me. 'A bit?'

So we're headed for our first round of assisted conception. I think for all women this must bring a mix of emotions: on the one hand, disappointment that you have to resort to this to make a baby; on the other hand, excitement that the baby you have been longing for might finally be made. The first step of the process for me and for many women is what is known as 'down-regulation'. This essentially involves shutting off your normal reproductive cycle so that your doctor can take control of it. It may involve an injection or a rather undignified nasal spray. Once down-regulation has been achieved you progress to the stage known as 'stimulation', which generally takes about two weeks. This involves daily injections designed to stimulate your ovaries to produce multiple follicles and therefore multiple eggs. The whole premise of IVF is that as well as assisting the fertilisation of egg and sperm by doing it outside the body, it also works to increase the probability of success by enabling a woman to produce many more eggs than she would normally release in a single month.

For the first week of our injections, Peter and I are away on holiday with a group of friends. We furtively administer the drugs in the privacy of our room, not telling anyone what we're up to. It feels rather like a childhood game of Doctors and Nurses. I can't help noticing that Peter seems to take particular pleasure in injecting me. As he draws the syringe and pushes the needle into my tummy, I close my eyes and think of George Clooney in *ER*…

During the second week of stimulation, we start to make regular trips to the clinic to see how my follicles are developing. Apparently this helps to pinpoint the right time to trigger ovulation, which involves another injection that has to be performed exactly thirty-six hours before my eggs are collected. Our doctor says that everything is progressing nicely.

The day of egg collection comes. We arrive at the clinic early. First up, we have to produce a sperm sample. The clinic has agreed that we can be together for this, and we are taken to a small room. This time we're not in a broom cupboard but it's still tiny. There's an incredibly uncomfortable-looking chair, which we avoid, and a hatch between the room and the lab from where we can hear the embryologists chatting about what they did over the weekend.

It takes us a long time. The more we worry about how long it's taking, the longer it takes. But we get there in the end and Peter heads to the lab with the little pot, promising me he won't lose sight of it. I am then taken through to a cubicle, told to get undressed and gowned up, and before I know it I'm lying on an operating table.

I've never had an operation in my life and everything is new to me. The room is filled with people who introduce themselves in turn. I'm rather touched that they've all turned out, just for me. There's our doctor, a nurse, an embryologist and the anaesthetist. (Ah, the anaesthetist, the man of my dreams. One of the great things about egg collection is the anaesthetic: it's the best sleep you'll ever have.)

Within seconds of getting settled, they've strapped a plastic mask to my face and I can feel myself going under. The next thing I know, I'm back in my cubicle coming round. I have no idea how they got me here. They must have picked me up off the operating trolley and carried through my leaden body, arm trailing on the ground. In my half-conscious state I immediately start to wonder whether they struggled to lift me and had to call in additional resources. I grimace at the embarrassment. Later I find out that they pushed me through on a trolley, but the space is so small, the corners so tight, I still don't quite understand how.

Peter is there when I wake up. It's so nice to see him. I feel as if I've been on a long journey and he's waiting at the arrivals gate to welcome me home. A nurse brings me a cup of tea and some biscuits. It's the best cup of tea and biscuits I've ever tasted.

I'm starting to like this IVF thing.

Then I remember our sperm. Peter assures me he's been with it the whole time and that as soon as I'm properly awake we can go round and see it. Half an hour later, sperm checked, we head out of the clinic for something to eat. It's a beautiful day and we wander over to Regent's Park and have lunch on the terrace of the café in the inner circle. It is as if we've just been through some sort of initiation ceremony and we've now moved on to the celebratory feast. It feels good to be alive, with all the possibilities that lie ahead.

After a couple of hours we are back at the clinic to witness the embryologist, Rob, injecting Peter's sperm into my eggs. We're taken through into the theatre where my eggs were collected earlier. It now feels eerily empty and quiet. Rob turns on a television monitor and then disappears into a side room. From here he talks us through the process as we watch what's happening on the screen. First he shows us Peter's sperm sample, with lots of tiny tadpole-like creatures swimming around. He chooses one of these at random, chops off its tail, which immediately paralyses it, and then sucks it up into a needle, with which he inserts it into one of my eggs. It's the most extraordinary thing to watch and, bizarrely, I actually start to feel lucky that we're conceiving a baby through IVF. Imagine being able to tell your children that you witnessed the moment when the sperm and egg that made them were first introduced. Incredible.

After each of my eggs has been injected, Rob carefully places them in an incubator that is heated to the exact temperature of the human body. He locks and seals the door, and promises that it won't be opened again until we come back tomorrow. As good as his word, the next day he breaks the seal and carefully removes them to see which have fertilised. Those that haven't are discarded and those that have are returned to the incubator, which is resealed. Rob assures us that they will not move again until they go back inside me. At this point I learn that today, the day after egg collection, is known as Day 1, and that the transfer of embryos generally takes place on Day 2, Day 3 or Day 5. (I forget to ask why they skip Day 4 – one to google later, I guess.)

In our case, on Day 3, they decide that it's already clear which of our embryos are the best quality. They photograph all of them and show us the two they have chosen to put back. One of them looks like it should be in a textbook. The picture shows six perfectly drawn circles shaped like the head of a flower, five around the outside and one in the middle. It's beautiful, and Rob tells us it's a grade one embryo – their top score. Result!

The transfer happens in the same room as egg collection. The procedure is relatively painless. It involves inserting a speculum – which looks rather like a classy piece of stainless steel cooking equipment – into my vagina and then using a long straw to transfer the embryos into my uterus. It doesn't take long and Peter is by my side.

As soon as the procedure is finished our doctor stands up, shakes our hands, wishes us the best of luck and leaves the room. It feels a bit abrupt, almost as if he's making a getaway. We look at each other, bemused, not quite sure what happens next. Ten minutes later a nurse comes in and tells us it's time to get dressed and go home. As we leave the clinic it feels as if we're newborn kittens: blinking in the sunlight, unsteady on our feet, we're stepping out alone into the world for the first time. Just us and our two embryos, on our own for the eponymous 'two-week wait'.

The 'two-week wait' is the name given to the time between your embryo transfer and your pregnancy test. You're pregnant but you're not pregnant, and it's impossible not to read every tiny twinge in your body as a positive sign. And then as a negative sign. I carry on working, as I have throughout my treatment. There are moments when I forget what is or isn't going on inside me. But there are times when I can't think of anything else.

I am due to do a pregnancy test on Tuesday at the clinic. They've given us the option of coming into the clinic for a blood test on Day 15 (post egg-collection) or waiting another day and doing it at home using an over-the-counter urine test. We've opted not to wait. On Saturday night, I notice I have a bit of light spotting. By Sunday morning the spotting hasn't gone away and, with Peter's encouragement, I call the clinic's out-of-hours emergency number. The nurse who answers the phone tells me, rather brusquely, that it's perfectly normal and not to worry.

By Monday morning the spotting has become heavier and redder, and by Tuesday I am bleeding. We make our way to the clinic with heavy hearts. They take some blood and ask us to wait. After half an hour a nurse calls us through to one of the consultation rooms.

'It's OK,' I say before she can say a word. 'We're prepared for the worst.'

'Well, it's not necessarily the worst,' she says. 'The test is inconclusive. We're going to have to send it off to an outside lab to double check. We'll be able to call you and let you know this afternoon.'

'How can it be inconclusive?' I ask.

'Well, the way that we confirm a pregnancy is by the presence of a hormone called HCG,' she explains. 'The hormone is released after an embryo has implanted into the lining of the womb, and can be detected either in your blood or in your urine. We can see that you do have some HCG in your blood, but the level looks low and we need to send it away to get a more exact measurement.' She pauses and looks at me. 'I understand it's hard, but everything may be fine. Let's just wait and see.'

'OK,' I say. 'I'm getting used to waiting. What's another couple of hours.'

Peter drives me back to work. My phone is by my side all afternoon. Like a ticking bomb it eventually goes off.

'Hello.'

'Is that Jessica?'

'Yes.'

'It's the clinic here. Can you just confirm your date of birth for me?'

'The twenty-first of the eleventh, 1970.'

'Sorry for the wait. I know you must be anxious.'

'A bit,' I say. 'Well, more than a bit.'

'I'm sure,' she says sympathetically. 'Well, we've got the results back but I'm afraid they're still inconclusive. The HCG level is sixteen, which means that the pregnancy hormone is definitely there, but at this stage we would expect it to be much higher. I'm afraid the only thing we can do is test you again in a couple of days and see whether the level has increased. In the first few weeks of pregnancy HCG generally doubles every forty-eight hours, so we'll have a much better indication of what's happening on Thursday.'

'Thursday?' I can't hide the despondency in my voice.

'Yes, Thursday. Would you be able to come into

the clinic that morning for another test?'

'I guess so,' I say flatly.

'I know this is difficult, Jessica, but try to stay positive. Everything may be OK.'

Try to stay positive. Everything may be OK. Two sentences that, in time, I would learn to loathe.

After two more days of hope and anxiety we head back to the clinic for another test, and another long wait. The phone rings.

'Hello.'

'Is that Jessica?'

'Yes.'

'It's the clinic here. Can you just confirm your date of birth for me?'

'The twenty-first of the eleventh, 1970.'

'I've got your results and I'm really sorry to have to say this but they're still inconclusive.'

'What? How?'

'Well, the HCG level has gone up. In fact it's doubled. It's now 36.7, but that's still much lower than we would expect at this stage.'

'I see,' I say. Not that I do. 'So what do we do now?'

'I'm afraid the only thing we can do is wait and keep monitoring it. It's clear that at least one of the embryos has implanted, but I'm afraid that it's unlikely, although not impossible, that the pregnancy is viable. We'd like you to come back in a week to test again.'

I put the phone down. I know it's no one's fault but I can't help feeling cheated. I was always aware of the risk that it might not work, but I had naively thought that, whatever happened, it would be a straightforward 'pregnant' or 'not pregnant'. I wasn't prepared for a situation where I seemed to be both 'pregnant' *and* 'not pregnant'. All the positivity we had felt at the beginning of the process becomes eclipsed by this uncertainty. Whilst there is still hope it feels too soon to be disappointed, but there doesn't seem much to be hopeful about either.

A week later we are back at the clinic. My HCG level still indicates that I am pregnant but it has dropped to 31.7. After another two weeks and another test it has dropped to below zero and, finally, it is officially confirmed that I am no longer pregnant. In medical terms, what has happened to me is known as a biochemical pregnancy. In layman's terms it's a very early miscarriage. If I had conceived naturally, I would probably never have known it had happened.

Your first round of failed IVF is an important milestone. It's the time when you become aware that, even with all the assistance medical science has to offer, this thing is not necessarily going to be easy to achieve. For me, it is also the first step in realising that all my paranoia about human fallibility is kind of irrelevant if the treatment doesn't actually work.

But there are also positive things to take from failure. You learn how your body reacts to treatment, and a good doctor will use this information next time. In our case, my body reacted well to the process. I had a good number of eggs, the majority of which fertilised. I had two high quality embryos put back on Day 3, and another four which were frozen. And at least one of my embryos implanted, resulting in the biochemical pregnancy. Our doctor assures us that these are all very good signs and a strong indication that, next time, things will work out well.

The Infertility Diaries Part IV

I feel a bit like I'm about to betray a secret in saying this, but your first round of IVF is the best – regardless of whether or not it gets you pregnant. It is a blissful time, when you are uninitiated in what will all too soon become emotionally draining obsessions. But that comes later. This is our first time and for now, at least, we are still innocent as cherubs.

TOP GIRLS

You have probably gathered by now that I work in a theatre. I'm not an actress, director or playwright. I oversee all the other stuff that goes into running a theatre: from looking after the money to making sure the loos are cleaned each morning.

I love my job and, if I'm honest, one of the things I love most about it is that whenever I'm at party and someone asks me what I do, they always say, 'What a great job!' It makes me feel proud and helps me to brace myself for the next question, which is usually: 'Do you have children?'

People often ask me how I got into working in the theatre. Like many people I started acting at school. I followed in the footsteps of Emma Thompson, who had acted on my school stage before me, but I was clever enough to realise that there wasn't an Oscar out there with my name on it. I was, however, very good at organising things and people (my friends would say bossy). I guess somewhere amongst all that is how it started.

I used to go to the theatre I run now on school trips as a child. I sometimes think of myself as a teenager all those years ago, sitting at the back of the upper circle, with no idea how important the building would become in my future.

I would never say that I'm good at my job, but I do work hard and try to be the best at it I can be. I think things are still difficult for women in senior roles. In my experience, even now, most people feel much more comfortable with a man in charge, and men are much more comfortable being in charge themselves (even those who are not very good at it).

When I first got my job, I remember an old boss of mine saying, 'Jessica, you're about to learn that it's tough at the top.' Sadly, the cliché is true. You quickly get used to the fact that part of your role is to be an organisational punch bag, and however hard you try, you can never please everyone all of the time. Power is undoubtedly seductive but it can also be lonely. Everybody looks to you to solve their problems but seldom ask if you have any of your own.

It is for this reason that I sidestep questions at work about whether I want children and haven't told anyone about our struggle with infertility. I go to great lengths to organise doctors' appointments at times when I can slip away unnoticed, and haven't taken any time off during our treatment. Even when I had my eggs collected under general anaesthetic in the morning, I was back at my desk by lunch. I tell myself that my strength and secrecy is another professional achievement but I am starting to wonder whether it is.

The Infertility Diaries Part V

The other day I jumped into a taxi and got chatting to the driver. I asked him the question I ask all (friendly) cabbies: which famous people have you picked up? He told me excitedly that last week he had picked up Emma Forbes – the one-time Saturday children's TV presenter and daughter of the actress Nanette Newman.

'She was my childhood crush,' he confided. 'It was very exciting.'

I smiled then said, 'Anyone else?'

'Well, one time, I picked up this guy…' he said. 'I asked him what he did for a living and he told me he was in a band. We liked a lot of the same stuff and had a long chat about music. Then, just before I dropped him off, I asked whether I'd have heard of the band he was in…'

'And had you?'

'You could say that…it was the Rolling Stones.'

I laughed.

'That's a brilliant story,' I said. 'Which one was it?'

'The drummer, Charlie Watts.'

'Oh, I wouldn't worry, nobody recognises drummers.'

He laughed back.

'That's what must be great about being a cab driver,' I continued. 'Meeting all sorts of people. Having conversations you would never otherwise have.'

'Yes,' he said. 'People tell me all sorts of things. I had

one woman the other day who told me all about going through IVF treatment. At the end of it she said, "I can't believe I told you all that."'

'I can,' I said. 'Sometimes there's no one else you can tell.'

The Curious Incident of the Spring Roll in the Night-Time

I pride myself on never being ill. In fifteen years of working I've never had a day off sick. Actually, that's not strictly true. I did once have a half-day when I had such bad tonsillitis I couldn't speak, but it was only a half-day, so I figure it doesn't count. Peter says it's not true that I don't get sick – it's just that when I do I go into denial. I admit that I do see sickness as a weakness, but I also seem to have been blessed with an invincible immune system. I'm just lucky (on that particular front), I guess.

It was therefore rather disheartening, not to mention embarrassing, when I started to suffer from regular attacks of indigestion. I know. Indigestion. Hardly the most street-cred condition. But, believe me, this was the sort of indigestion that laughed in the face of a packet of Rennie. It would come on at night, last for hours, and occasionally cause multiple bouts of vomiting. Nice.

Oddly, the first time I experienced these symptoms was whilst undergoing my initial round of IVF. Midway through my two-week wait I woke up in the middle of the night with a piercing pain in my chest that lasted several hours. Thereafter, these night-time visitations started to occur sporadically. There wasn't any obvious pattern. I could go for weeks without one and then three would come at once. I went to my GP, who sent me to the hospital for some tests. They couldn't find anything. It was a mystery.

At our follow-up appointment at the fertility clinic, we ask our doctor whether he knows of any link between IVF and indigestion. He doesn't. In fact, he assures us that the two things are completely unrelated and recommends we undertake a cycle of IVF using our frozen embryos in a couple of months' time.

'Do you think your indigestion could be stress-related?' Peter says as we're walking back to the car.

'I don't feel stressed,' I say.

'What does stress feel like?'

I glare at him. 'Stress is not an illness. It's a mindset.'

'In that case I'm glad I don't have your mind.'

We get in the car and Peter starts the engine.

'Don't you think you should talk to someone about what we're going through?' he says. 'It might help.'

'I talk to you, don't I?'

'But wouldn't it be good to get another perspective? I'm sure it can't be helping holding it all inside. Maybe it's the tension that's giving you indigestion.'

'Maybe.'

I don't know if I'm not convinced or just reluctant to admit the possibility that I might not be coping.

'I understand why you don't feel you can tell anyone at work' Peter continues. 'And I know you don't want your mum to worry about you. But you're not talking about it to any of your friends either. I thought that's what girls do. Talk about stuff.'

'They do, but this is different.'

'Why?'

'Most of my friends are having babies. Infertility is a kind of conversation show-stopper.'

Over the next few days I think about what Peter has said. Maybe I should talk to someone. Maybe I could talk to Beth. It is now well over a year since our evening out at the Railway Tavern when she announced that she and Thomas were about to start trying for a baby. Unlike so many of our other school friends, she still hasn't got pregnant either. It's not something we've talked about much, but whenever we see each other I know there's a silent acknowledgement that we're both still baby-less.

A few days later I decide to give her a call and arrange to meet up.

'So can I ask how the baby-making's going?' I say as we settle into the coffee-shop sofas with two cups of peppermint tea. We're both displaying the universal symbol of women trying to conceive: withdrawal from caffeine.

'It's not,' she says. 'My period started this morning.'

'Ovulation predictor kit failed again?'

'Yup. Every time.'

'I recently read somewhere that sex never gets back to normal after the tyranny of the ovulation predictor kit.'

'God, that's a deeply depressing thought.'

'So have you been to see a doctor?' I ask.

'Yes – we've had the tests but they haven't thrown anything up. We're due to start this thing called IUI next month.'

'I've had that.'

'You have?'

'It's a long story, but suffice to say it was a disaster.' I take a sip of tea. 'You'd better tell Thomas to prepare himself for the horror of the "producing room".'

'It's OK. We've got that one covered,' she says. 'They've said we can bring the sample with us as long as we get there within thirty minutes and keep it warm.'

'That's a result.'

'They've suggested I put it between my breasts.'

'I suspect Freud would have something to say about that.'

She laughs.

'And how are things going for you and Peter?'

'We've just done our first round of IVF. It didn't work.'

'Oh Jess, I'm so sorry. I had no idea.'

'To be honest, no one does. Telling people just felt like an added pressure.'

'I know what you mean. Especially as everyone else seems to find it so easy.'

'Exactly.'

We look at each other. A moment of shared understanding that doesn't need any other words.

'So how's Peter feeling about it all?'

'We avoid talking about it most of the time, but I think he's probably worried.'

'About what?'

'About me; about what happens if it doesn't work; about how much it's costing; about the possibility that he'll never be able to have another drink again without me looking at him disapprovingly…'

'As if relationships weren't hard enough already.'

We are both silent for a moment.

'It's good to see you, Beth,' I say.

'It's good to talk,' she replies.

I set down my cup and turn to her.

'Shall we have a coffee?'

'That's a bit reckless, isn't it?' she laughs.

'Sometimes you need to say, "Fuck it, right now I need a double-shot cappuccino more than I need a baby."'

'You're right. And let's have a slice of cake too.'

'I bet cake's banned.'

'Everything's banned these days.'

'So let's start a revolution!'

A few months later Peter and I go through a frozen IVF cycle using the remaining embryos from our initial round of treatment. This proves to be far less intense than the first time and simply involves shutting down my natural cycle, taking some drugs to create the right environment within my uterus, and then popping the fertilised eggs back. All four of our frozen embryos survive the thawing process, but as only two can be transferred we have to say goodbye to the others. Some things aren't different about the process though. Firstly, there's another two-week wait to contend with (nor is it any easier this time around). And secondly, we end up with the same result as last time – although, thankfully, the uncertainty is less prolonged. The first blood test indicates that I am pregnant but the HCG level is low. Two days later the level has dropped. Another biochemical pregnancy.

Again our doctor says that, whilst this is disappointing, it is still a good sign. He encourages us to undergo another full round of IVF as soon as possible. His advice is that we simply replicate everything we did last time. As I responded so well, there's no reason to do anything differently. So we do. I down-regulate, take the same dosage of stimulation drugs, and turn up for egg collection in eager anticipation of another anaesthetic. What I don't know, as I breezily enter the clinic saying 'hello' to the now familiar receptionist, is that I'm about to learn two of the most important lessons of IVF: firstly, that no two rounds are ever the same; and secondly, that the happy ignorance of your first round will never be repeated.

When I come round from the anaesthetic, Peter is sitting waiting for me. I don't feel quite as refreshed as I did last time, and the tea and bourbon biscuits don't taste quite as good.

A nurse comes through to check on me.

'Well done, Jessica,' she says. 'You did really well. We collected nine eggs.'

'Nine?' I say.

'That's right.'

'Didn't I have more last time?'

'I'm not sure, I haven't got your records here. But there's nothing to worry about. Nine is good, very good.'

The next day we go into the clinic, just as before, to see how many eggs have fertilised and watch them being moved into new Petri dishes. Of my nine eggs, four have achieved fertilisation. At face value, nothing to worry about here either. But – and it's a big but – a new chapter in my IVF journey has begun.

Last time, the first time, I didn't pay any attention to egg numbers and fertilisation rates. I had sixteen eggs; thirteen fertilized; two embryos were transferred on Day 3; four more were of good enough quality to be frozen. As far as I knew, this was what happened to everyone. Even if it didn't, it was what happened to me.

So why are things so different this time around? We did everything exactly the same. The only change was that I had a bit of acupuncture and took some supplements prescribed by a very chi-chi clinic that promotes natural therapies alongside conventional IVF. Surely this should have helped, not hindered the process.

I do feel ungrateful saying this. I'm sure some women have to face a situation where they produce no eggs at all or they do but none of them fertilises. Whilst it is significantly fewer than last time, we are still lucky enough to have four embryos, and although two of them don't survive much beyond the second day, the other two are put back on Day 3. But as we go home to start our third two-week wait, I have this sinking feeling that, whatever happens this time around, my relationship with IVF is never going to be quite the same again.

When we get home, we decide to treat ourselves to a Chinese takeaway and an evening of trash TV – heaven, apart from the absence of a glass of red wine. We go to bed, tired and happy. Peter kisses my tummy and says goodnight to our babies on their first night at home with Mum and Dad.

In the middle of the night I wake up with a pain in my chest. Indigestion.

'Hello,' I think. 'Why now?'

It is at least a month since my last attack and I have almost forgotten the dull, unrelenting ache. I lie still with my eyes shut, trying to pretend it isn't there, but after a while the sickness starts. I run to the bathroom and retch: a case of last night's Chinese takeaway revisited. I crawl back to bed and lie on my back with my knees up. Then on my front in child's pose. Then on my side hugging a cushion.

Nothing is comfortable. Nothing will relieve it. I run to the loo again. More Chinese with a bit of leftover lunch mixed in. I go into the sitting room and turn on the television to try to distract myself from the pain. It doesn't work. I'm sick again, this time barely getting to the loo in time.

After a couple of hours Peter suggests we walk round the block. The cool night air is refreshing but the movement just shifts the pain; I bend over and throw up in the gutter. I must look like I'm on my way home from a good night out. If only.

We go back home to bed. It's starting to get light and usually things would be easing off by now. Four hours of agony is generally my maximum sentence. But the pain and sickness is showing no sign of subsiding, even though my stomach is empty and all I have to offer up is canary-yellow bile. Peter has to go to work and I insist that I'll be all right on my own. It's a Saturday so at I least I don't have to go into the office myself. When he gets home in the evening I'm still in bed. The pain and sickness has finally gone but I am utterly exhausted.

A few days before I am due to do my pregnancy test, I start spotting. The day after that I start bleeding. I don't even bother to take a test. I can't believe anything would have survived that first night of indigestion and sickness anyway. What's the point?

The Infertility Diaries Part VI

As soon as your friends start having babies, and you don't, your relationship changes. They want to talk about sleeping patterns; how long to breastfeed; whether to Gina Ford or not to Gina Ford. It's not that I find these conversations upsetting, or that I'm not interested (although these subjects aren't particularly interesting if you don't have children). I just don't know how to have them. So after a while you stop getting invited round to dinner, and you stop inviting them. Then you realise that your friends have made some new friends – friends who all have babies too.

THE 100M HURDLE RACE

The IVF process is like the 100m hurdle race, but with six huge hurdles instead of ten. At every stage you can only see the hurdle directly in front of you, but as each one is cleared, the finishing line, with its definitive ribbon of success or failure, gets closer.

Hurdle 1: How many follicles?

The first hurdle is how your body responds to stimulation. The aim is to develop a decent number of follicles of a similar size in each ovary. You're always anxious prior to the first scan. What if there are only a couple of big ones and the rest are tiny? What if there aren't any follicles at all? During stimulation the number of follicles becomes your first daily obsession.

Hurdle 2: How many eggs?

Soon the number of follicles becomes irrelevant; now the important question is how many eggs? Not every follicle will release an egg, and not every egg released will be mature. As soon as you wake up from the anaesthetic after egg collection, it's the first question you ask. It's a numbers game: the more the better.

Hurdle 3: How many fertilised?

The morning after egg collection is the next hurdle: how many eggs have fertilised? In IVF it's rarely, if ever, 100 per cent, which is why you need a good number of follicles and then a good number of eggs in order to increase your chances of success. Today everything that's happened over the previous two weeks no longer matters. This is now regarded as Day 1; you're halfway through, just three more hurdles to jump.

Hurdle 4: Days 2 to 5

Over the next few days your embryos begin cell division and all you can do is watch and wait. As each day passes some will progress, others will falter and fail. From Day 2 of your embryos' life they start to be graded, and this influences the decision as to which ones should be put back when. In the UK, currently, if you're under forty you can have two embryos back; and over forty, three embryos. As soon as it becomes clear which embryos are the best – or maybe they are the only embryos you have – your clinic will want to put them back where they belong. If you have produced a small number of eggs, it becomes clear pretty quickly which to put back. If you have produced a larger number and all of them are developing nicely, they are likely to hang on to see which embryos develop into blastocysts. This is the term used for embryo development on Day 5. In theory, an embryo that becomes a blastocyst has the best chance of survival, but the embryos will only be cultured to this stage if there are more than a few good ones of similar quality.

Hurdle 5: The two-week wait

The penultimate hurdle is the dreaded two-week wait: the period between your embryo transfer and pregnancy test, when time seems interminable. You become hyper-aware of every twinge, or lack of twinge, in your body, oscillating between thinking it's a good sign, then thinking it must be bad. Every physical movement or negative emotion feels like it might have jeopardised the process. You know that being positive is important, but you also don't trust yourself to deliver.

Hurdle 6: The pregnancy test

And finally, the test itself, when all that stands between you and happiness is a double line. But having longed for the wait to be over, you now wish it could continue. After all, there's no guarantee of a medal at the end of this race, and to prolong doubt is to prolong hope.

The Infertility Diaries Part VII

Infertility has ruined the beautiful relationship I had with alcohol, my perfect partner at the end of a hard day's work. These days our dealings have become uneasy. I am suspicious of whether it is affecting my fertility. I am even more suspicious of the affair it may be having with Peter. Yet, at the same time, I'm grateful for its ability to numb the pain; to make the world seem an infinitely more survivable place. But then I start to resent it, knowing that reality and regret always follow later. I long for something else to come along that will force me to walk out on the relationship – just a trial separation of nine months would do. Maybe then we can rekindle our love again.

DREAMING SPIRES

It's time for a change. For the last few years we have been living in a series of one-bedroom flats in different parts of London, and I am starting to become obsessed with the idea of buying a house and having our own front door. We start spending our Saturdays trawling around estate agents. I realise it's probably some form of baby-displacement activity.

It's the height of the property market and it soon becomes clear that the only houses we can afford are in neighbourhoods on the outskirts of London, which are full of thirty-something couples and their Maclaren buggies. I want a house but I can't bear the thought of being the odd couple, so, in a moment of reckless spontaneity, we buy a house in Oxford. Not that there's anything wrong or reckless about Oxford per se. A house there is certainly cheaper than its counterpart in London and, according to the UK's property oracle (aka Kirsty and Phil), it's a good investment as it will always be rentable to students (and rich students at that). Nevertheless, it is a bit of a weird thing to do when you don't know anyone else who lives there. And you work in London.

But there is another reason. I have been going through a tough time at work. I'm spending an increasing number of hours at my desk, regularly coming in with the cleaners at six in the morning and not leaving until past ten at night. I am also going in at weekends, which, along with workaholics everywhere, I tell myself is the *only* time I can get anything done. Peter keeps nagging me that this can't be helping our attempts to conceive. I know he's probably right and that I'm using work to numb the pain of not having a baby. We both hope that a move to Oxford might be a good, if slightly drastic, way to force me to change my work–life balance.

As soon as our offer is accepted I ring Beth to tell her. She has now been through several rounds of IUI. All negative. She is on the NHS waiting list for her first round of IVF.

'I've got some news,' I say.

'Really?' she says excitedly.

'Not that sort of news,' I say quickly. 'We've bought a house.'

'You have? Where?'

'Oxford.'

A moment's silence.

'Where?' she says again.

'Oxford.'

'That's what I thought you said. Why?'

'It seemed like a good idea.'

'What about work? Are you going to commute?'

'That's the plan.'

'At least you won't be tempted to go in at weekends any more.'

'That too.'

She's silent again. She seems to be processing the information.

'Do you know anyone there?'

'Not a soul.'

'But you'll meet people,' she says. 'It's exciting.' Her voice sounds genuine, if a bit cautious.

'It is,' I say. 'A new start is just what we need. Anyway, how are things with you? Got any news about your IVF yet?'

'No...but I do have some news...'

She is hesitant, and I feel a familiar crumpling in my chest as I realise what she's about to say. Why isn't there a word in the English language for feeling happy for someone and sad for yourself at the same time?

Shortly after we move into our new house, we decide it's time for a change of clinic too. Over the last two years we have been through four failed attempts at IVF there (rounds one and two which resulted in biochemical pregnancies; round three being the indigestion episode; and a fourth round in which I also started spotting and then bleeding before test day and was negative). As much as I love the staff there, it feels like the end of a relationship, when you both still care about each other but instinct tells you that it's not going to work out in the long term and it's time to move on.

The first thing we do is sign up with a new GP in Oxford. When I go for my registration appointment, I am seen by a friendly male doctor. He asks me about my general health and I give him a brief summary of the last few years.

He listens attentively.

'I realise how hard it must be,' he says. 'I really do. My wife and I have been through infertility treatment ourselves.'

'You have?' I say.

'Yes. If you're thinking about going to a new clinic there are a couple that I would recommend. One of them is here in Oxford, based at the John Radcliffe Hospital. It takes both NHS and private patients. It worked for us.'

I can hardly believe his candidness or his kindness. A lot of GPs are rather aloof and uncomfortable around the subject of infertility. It is so comforting finally to find one who is open and clearly wants to help.

A few weeks later I bump into him in the supermarket on a Saturday morning, two beautiful children hanging off his shopping trolley. I smile tentatively, not really expecting him to remember who I am.

'Hello,' he says.

'Hi – I'm one of your patients,' I say, just for clarification.

'I remember,' he says. And then more quietly, almost conspiratorially, as he nods towards his children: 'See, it can work.'

Sadly, I never saw that doctor again. A few months later he left the practice for a new job. But in that moment – a chance encounter between two almost strangers in a busy supermarket aisle – there was a profound sense of connection and understanding. I made up my mind. Our next clinic would be the Fertility Unit at the John Radcliffe Hospital.

So maybe there is another reason we moved to Oxford. Maybe these dreaming spires are meant to lead us to our longed-for child.

Our first appointment is with their consultant gynaecologist, a softly spoken, charismatic Irishman who has recently been listed in a weekend newspaper supplement as one of the most successful fertility doctors in the country. We talk openly about our treatment to date. He says that in his opinion our previous clinic is very good, and that it probably won't be possible for his practice to facilitate the same level of witnessing as we had there. At least he's honest. He also says that everything about the response and results of our treatment to date indicate that we should try again, and that we have a very strong chance of success. We like his style and decide to embark on another, our fifth, round of IVF.

Things go pretty well. I don't reach the dizzy heights of egg numbers and fertilisation rates that I did on our first round, but it's better than our recent tries and, on Day 3, I get some exciting news. The clinic calls to say that five of our embryos are still developing really nicely and they are going to wait to see which become blastocysts and put them back on Day 5.

Rightly or wrongly, the blastocyst has become my Holy Grail. Statistics indicate that embryos which are transferred on Day 5, when they have reached this developmental stage, are the most likely to implant and go on to achieve a successful pregnancy. In fact, some doctors say – but this is not something that is commonly acknowledged or practised – that it is not worth putting embryos back before Day 5 because, unless they reach this stage in the lab, it is very unlikely that they will form a viable pregnancy. Until now I have always had my transfer on Day 3, so to be going beyond this feels like a mini-triumph. It also gives my body a few more days to recover from egg collection and, in my mind, for our embryos to grow stronger before they are unleashed in the hostile environment I'm starting to think my womb must be. By Day 5 four of our embryos have developed into good quality blastocysts, so two are transferred and the other two are frozen.

This time around our two-week wait is during August, coinciding with the Edinburgh Festival which Peter and I both attend every year for work. The familiar smell of hops that fills the city hits me as we get out of the taxi on George Street. It feels good to be back in one of the most beautiful cities in the world, never better than during festival time (although a fair few Scots might disagree). I think about our embryos, snuggling down inside me, protected from the biting Scottish summer. I am looking forward to the day when we'll be here together as a family and I'll have a proper excuse for us to spend hours watching street theatre – something Peter never allows me to do now.

I persuade our hotel receptionist to give us a room on one of the highest floors (always my first choice for hotel rooms on account of the views). We hit the jackpot with one that overlooks Edinburgh Castle – here's hoping we're on to a lucky streak. Over the next few days I hare round the city seeing shows. I love festival theatregoing. For someone who regularly falls asleep in the theatre at the end of a long day, there's nothing better than a play in the morning with a coffee and a croissant. It is also a great way of taking my mind off the two-week wait. That is, until the now all-too-familiar curse of pre-test spotting begins. After each show I make a beeline for the ladies' loo to check on the situation. At first it's a very light pink and almost ignorable. But within forty-eight hours it gets darker and redder. I'm practically bleeding and there's no mistaking it.

Peter persuades me to the ring the clinic. I hardly see the point but eventually comply.

'I'm on my two-week wait and have started spotting,' I say. 'I don't know why I'm ringing, really. I know there's nothing you can do.'

'When are you due to test?'

(At our new clinic they give you a urine test to do at home and don't give you the option of an early blood test.)

'In a few days' time.'

'It's important that you do the test. Spotting is common…'

'I know,' I say. 'You're going to tell me that I should try to stay positive. Everything might be OK.'

'That's exactly right,' the nurse says encouragingly.

'Except I know it isn't OK. I know it hasn't worked.'

'You may feel that, but it is still really important that you take the test and ring us with the result.'

'Fine, I'll take the test, but why don't you just write on my notes now that it's negative and save me the call. If by any miracle it's positive, I'll let you know.' I sound cross but I don't care.

'I'm afraid I can't do that. You need to ring us

with the result when you've taken the test.' She is starting to sound irritated too.

'Well that's stupid,' I say. 'And unnecessarily painful.'

I hang up the phone. It isn't one of my finest conversations.

I spend most of the next few days sitting by the window of our hotel room, looking out at the castle. There are a growing number of uncollected tickets waiting for me at box offices across the city. I venture out cautiously for the shows I have to go to for work, crossing the street whenever I see someone I know to avoid conversation.

On the final night of the festival, as I sit in our room, fireworks exploding over the castle, flooding Edinburgh in multicoloured light, I decide to do the test to prove what I already know.

I'm right: it's negative. I ring the clinic the next morning to tell them.

OUT DAMNED SPOT

For the first few days there's nothing.
You don't look.
You don't even think about looking.

Then, suddenly, a sign.
Faint at first.
Almost unnoticeable. Almost a surprise.

After that you start to look.
Dabbing for a few seconds longer than you need.
Peering intently.

In the beginning it's a light salmon pink.
Such a pretty, unoffending colour.
You google 'implantation bleeding'.
   Persuade yourself that this is it.

A few hours pass. A day perhaps.
The pink continues.
Sometimes very visible. Sometimes less so.

And then something dark brown.
Small, solid, string-like.
You google 'implantation bleeding' again.
   Persuade yourself that this is it.

Now you dab a little harder.
Really push around.
The pink is darker than it was, tinged with rust.

Then nothing.
No sign at all.
For a whole afternoon. A night, even.

Now you wipe more softly. Almost imperceptibly.
Just to prove that you're right.
That it's gone.

You start to feel positive.
You re-check the absence frequently.
Then leave it a little longer.

But then the salmon pink is back.
And suddenly, a streak of carmine red.
You google 'bleeding in early pregnancy'.
    Read that it is relatively common.

Then another streak of red. And another.
Unavoidable. Undeniable.
You know nothing can survive it. That the end of
    hope is near.

It doesn't matter how many times I'm told:
Stay positive. Everything may be OK.
I don't believe it.

I am Lady Macbeth. Guilty as charged.

The Infertility Diaries Part VIII

I'm mentoring a teenager at work who is participating in one of our theatre projects for disadvantaged young people. She's seventeen and has spent most of her life in care. As we sit and chat I can't help noticing that she's got scars on the inside of her arms where she's cut herself. I know I should feel sorry for her; I know how privileged I am. But all I feel is jealousy. She's seventeen. And pregnant.

WHAT A DIFFERENCE A DAY MAKES

It is six weeks since our first round of IVF at the clinic in Oxford. Our running total now stands at one frozen and four full cycles, with nothing to show for any of them. We are due to attend the clinic in a couple of days for a debrief and to work out what to do next.

For some reason I haven't had another period since our last round of treatment. I'm not unduly worried, as it is relatively common with IVF for your menstrual cycle to take a while to get back to normal. However, this never happened on my previous cycles so it's been playing on my mind. I keep thinking about it, then pushing it away, but that night, on my way to dinner with a friend, I walk past Boots and suddenly find myself at the counter buying a pregnancy test.

Getting your sex life back to normal after a round of failed fertility treatment is never easy. It's one of the last things you feel like doing and you start to wonder what the point is anyway. Thinking back over the last six weeks, I recall that Peter and I have made love once, but only once. I know it's mad to think that I might be pregnant but, as I am staying over with my parents in London, I tell myself that I can do the test without telling him. Then, when it's negative, I can stop thinking about it and get on with deciding what we're going to do next.

The following morning I wake up early and reach for the test in my bag. I feel stupid doing this, but keep assuring myself that nobody needs to know. I tear off the cellophane around the box with my teeth and take out the instructions. Read them carefully. Read them again. Then I get up and go quietly into the bathroom to pee on the stick.

Back in bed, I hold the test out in front of me. There is a clear vertical red line in the circular control box on the right, showing that the test has worked. There is another vertical red line in the square box on the left and, within just a few minutes, it is bisected by a horizontal red line. I look at the instructions again. Pregnant? Me? For a few minutes I sit there, incredulous. After years of having sex to schedule and five failed attempts at IVF, could I really have got pregnant from one night when I wasn't even trying?

I reach for my phone, hold it out in front of the stick, and take a photograph. Even on camera the red cross is clearly visible. Then I call Peter. He answers within a couple of rings.

'Peter, are you lying down?

'Sleeping actually. It's 6 a.m. What else do you think I'm doing?'

'Good, because this is going to come as a shock. I think I'm pregnant.'

'What?' He suddenly sounds awake.

'My period should have started by now and it hasn't. I just thought I'd do a test to make sure before we see the doctor tomorrow. And it's positive.'

'Why haven't you said anything before?'

'I didn't want you to think I was getting my hopes up for nothing. I was just so sure it would be negative. But it's not. Hang up the phone; I'll send you the photograph to prove it.'

The rest of the day passes in a haze. I am in my office, working as normal, and then suddenly remember and snatch a look at the stick in my bag. The cross is starting to fade but it is definitely there. Every time I look at it I feel a rush of excited gratitude.

On the way home that evening I buy another test. We've agreed to do it in the morning before going to the clinic. Just to make sure. It's like the night before Christmas. I can hardly sleep.

At 4.30 a.m. I nudge Peter.

'Can I do it now?'

'OK. Put the light on,' he says.

It is clear that he hasn't been able to sleep either. I reach over for the test, which I placed carefully on my bedside table last night, get up and go into the bathroom. I purposefully avoid looking at the stick when I've peed on it but come back to bed and hand it straight to Peter.

'You decide,' I say.

'How long does it take?'

'Up to three minutes.'

'And what am I looking for?'

'A red cross in the box on the left.'

'Done deal,' he says. 'I can see it already.'

Our appointment at the clinic is at 2 p.m. Unusually, I have a work meeting in Oxford that morning. I'm late and dash out of the house without having had any breakfast – not very sensible for a newly pregnant woman, I know, but some habits are hard to break. Especially double ones – in my case being late *and* skipping breakfast.

Towards the end of my meeting I start feeling a bit faint, so, as soon as it finishes, I decide to head over to the café in the church beside the magnificent Radcliffe Camera for something to eat. It is one of those beautiful sunny autumn days which always makes me think of Oxford as England's Florence. As I make my way through the cobbled streets I start to feel dizzy and am relieved to arrive at the café and sit down. I call Peter to explain where I am and he offers to pick me up in the car. He's cross with me for not eating and, for once, I accept that I may need to start thinking for two and, at the very least, eating for one.

When I finish my sandwich I pop to the loo before heading out to meet him. I don't give it a moment's thought so it comes as a bit of a shock to see a smear of light pink on the toilet tissue. I've had no sign of a period for weeks. Then a positive pregnancy test. Now I'm spotting. I knew it was too good to be true.

Peter is waiting for me in the car outside the

King's Arms, just across the square. He takes the news quietly.

'Please don't tell me to stay positive and that it might be fine,' I say. 'Spotting is not a good sign. It's never a good sign.'

'OK, I won't,' he says. 'But let's wait and see what the doctor has to say.'

We drive to the clinic in silence. They have recently moved premises to a new building in the middle of a business park on the edge of town. It seems such an odd place to have a fertility clinic. The new building has had a lot of money spent on it. It has clearly been interior-designed. The colours are all oranges and lime greens. It looks as if the team from one of those TV makeover shows has come in.

Our doctor takes us through to one of the consultation rooms. The wallpaper is a contemporary version of William Morris: metallic with a floral swirl. The room is empty apart from a table, three chairs and a contemporary standard lamp.

'So, Jessica…Peter…I'm really sorry about the outcome,' he starts, 'but I have to say that in IVF terms this was a really positive cycle. Seven eggs fertilised. Four achieved really nice blastocysts –'

'Sorry…' I say, 'I mean I'm sorry to interrupt, but before you go any further we need to let you know something that has happened over the last few days.'

He stops. 'Yes?'

'Well, the cycle was definitely negative. I started bleeding before the test date but I still did a test and it was negative. But I haven't had another period since and it's now nearly six weeks. So yesterday, just to rule out the possibility that we might have got pregnant naturally this month, I did a test, and it was positive. We did another one today. It was positive again. Then an hour ago I started spotting so…' I pause to draw breath, 'before you go any further, I'm hoping you can tell us what's going on, because something definitely is.'

I stop to breathe again.

'Well,' he says calmly. 'We'd better do a scan and find out.'

He shows us into a room across the hallway and leaves me to get undressed. After a few minutes there is a soft knock at the door. Peter squeezes my hand. Then the doctor comes in and turns the lights out. He stares at the screen intently as he moves the scanning probe around inside me.

'Does this hurt?' he asks.

'No.'

'What about this?'

'No.'

'And this?'

'No.'

'It doesn't hurt at all?'

'No. Not really.'

'OK. Get dressed and go back into the consultation room. I'll meet you in there.'

And with that he gets up and leaves the room.

Peter and I wait in tense silence for him to return. At least ten minutes pass.

'Why is he taking so long?' I whisper.

Then the door clicks. He comes in and sits down. He looks how I imagine doctors look when they have to give bad news.

'It's bad news, isn't it?' I say.

'I'm afraid so,' he says slowly. 'You are pregnant. But I believe the pregnancy is ectopic, which means that the embryo has implanted outside the womb. You're going to have to have an operation to remove it. I've already called the hospital; they're expecting you. You need to go there straight away.'

It is difficult to take it all in. I don't know what I thought he was going to say, but it certainly wasn't this. My mind immediately turns to work.

'An operation? That means I'll have to have time off work. How much time?'

'It's difficult to tell at this stage, but at least two weeks, maybe more.'

'Two weeks,' I exclaim. 'I've never had two weeks off work.' And then, more quietly: 'I can't believe after everything we've been through that I get pregnant naturally and this happens.'

'I very much doubt it has happened this month,' he says. 'It is much more likely that this pregnancy is the result of the IVF.'

'But I don't understand,' I say. 'The test was negative. More to the point, that would mean I'm nearly three months pregnant.'

'Yes,' he says. 'Which is why you have to go to the hospital right away. This is potentially a very dangerous situation.'

It's funny how you can go for years hiding the truth about something and then in an unexpected second it all starts to unravel.

I call work on the way to the hospital. I open my mouth to explain but all I can get out is: 'I'm not going to make it into work today…I'm on my way to the hospital…I'm sorry…' my voice starts to shake uncontrollably. 'I think I'm going to have to pass you over to Peter now…'

I hand over the phone. His voice is clear and calm. It's as if he's talking about someone else. I feel like I'm outside my body, looking down on us both. I can't believe this is happening.

Then he rings my mum. I can hear her shocked concern at the end of the line. I know she's been longing for me to give her a grandchild but neither of us has officially broached the subject, not wanting to put pressure on the other. Of course, not saying anything hasn't taken the pressure away.

When we arrive at the gynaecological wing of the hospital there is the inevitable wait. After a while I am called through for a blood test to confirm the pregnancy and see what level my hormones are. This is followed by another long wait. The results come back positive. The HCG pregnancy hormone is in the several thousands. I think back to my biochemical pregnancies, when I spent days willing it to increase beyond double figures. The irony is painful. The nurse informs us that they will operate early tomorrow.

It is the first time I've spent the night in a hospital and, despite being in shock, I also find it a bit exciting. I am given a bed with my own personal TV; a green NHS gown; and I'm rather touched by the care they take in checking my blood pressure every few hours right the way through the night. But it is also a profoundly sad experience, and not just because I am there to terminate a pregnancy that I have longed for. It highlights how isolated I have become by telling so few people about what I am going through, and by moving to Oxford where we don't know anyone and it's difficult for friends and family just to drop by. Peter is my main source of support and my only visitor.

The following morning I am taken in for surgery. The anaesthetist asks me to count down from ten to one and, the next thing I know, I am coming round in the recovery room. There's no tea, biscuits or Peter, and although I keep asking the nurses if I can see him, he doesn't appear. Eventually they take me back to the ward. He isn't there either.

'Do you know where my partner is?' I ask one of the nurses.

'I think he's in the waiting room,' she says. 'I'll go and get him.'

Finally, Peter emerges around the curtain of my cubicle, looking concerned.

'How are you?' he asks.

'Better for seeing you,' I say. My voice still sounds woozy. 'I kept asking for you but they wouldn't get you.'

'I kept asking for you,' he says. 'You've been gone over four hours. I was going out of my mind with worry.'

Later that afternoon my surgeon comes to check on me during his rounds.

'How are you feeling?' he asks.

'OK, I think.'

'You will probably feel very tired; you were asleep for quite a while.'

'Why was that? Peter said I was gone for four hours.'

'Well, we had quite a bit of difficulty finding the foetus. Usually with ectopic pregnancies it is in one of the fallopian tubes, but in your case it wasn't in either of them.'

'It wasn't?'

'No. It was in your stomach.'

'My stomach? How did it get there?'

'It must have passed from the womb, up through the fallopian tubes and then down into the abdomen. It is highly unusual though.'

As soon as he's gone I google 'ectopic pregnancy' on my phone. Apparently they most commonly occur when the embryo implants in a fallopian tube on its way down to the uterus, but in rare cases they can implant in all sorts of places. I read about one woman who had an abdominal ectopic and actually carried her baby to term, although it was born very prematurely. I can't help wishing this had been me but I know that's stupid. Stupid and dangerous.

My second and third nights in hospital are not as much fun as the first. I'm walking like an old woman, carrying a bag full of blood that seems to be attached to my stomach (to be honest, I don't look too closely). Peter stays for as long as he can on the day of the operation, but he has to go to a work event that evening and it's not something he can easily get out of. I imagine him having to make polite conversation, exchanging the usual pleasantries about the weather. The juxtaposition of public and private is something that has always fascinated me. How we never really know what's going on in other people's lives. How most of the time we never ask or say.

I am on a ward with three other women. I have no idea what each of them is in for, except that this is an antenatal ward and everyone is in for something baby-related. The woman in the bed next to me looks very sick. She sleeps a lot. There are two other women at the end of the ward. They are both pregnant but are experiencing complications and have been admitted for observation. They talk constantly about the intricacies of their pregnancies. It's hard listening to it. I know there's always a shortage of hospital beds but surely there must be a better way of managing this?

On Sunday morning I am discharged. Although I've only been in hospital for a few days it suddenly feels quite a wrench to leave. It's amazing how quickly you become institutionalised.

My surgeon comes to see me one last time before I go.

'I advise you to take a minimum of two weeks off before you go back to work,' he says. 'Shall I write you a sick note?'

'No, it's OK,' I say. 'The only person at work who will deny me any sick leave is myself.'

He laughs.

Peter picks me up from the hospital and drives us home. The house feels like it does when you come back from a holiday: strange and unlived-in. I can't settle. Peter has to go away for work for a few days so I decide to go with him and stay at the hotel where he's been booked a room. In many ways it's serendipitous. There's nothing quite as comforting as the fresh white sheets and daily towel change of a good hotel.

For three days straight I don't leave the hotel. But within a week I'm back at work.

The Infertility Diaries Part IX

Public holidays are hard. Especially Christmas. I long to experience the excitement of the family going out to buy the tree and decorating it to the sound of cheesy Christmas classics; of baking biscuits and stirring the pudding; of buying stocking presents and opening them together in bed on Christmas morning. This year we've decided to go away. Somewhere hot. Somewhere we're not reminded of the family we haven't got.

SOCKS AND STAIRS

I've always admired couples who say they never argue. Peter and I get cross with each other all the time. If there's a reason to take offence, one of us invariably will. We then begin a game of football, passing the ball of anger back and forth, scoring whenever we can. I know some people say there's passion in disagreement, that hurt is better out than in. But it would be nice. Not to argue. About even the smallest things.

These are some of the things that make me cross about Peter:

When I ask him to do something, he always says later.

He never says no to a drink. Or two.

When he puts on a pair of blue socks with a black suit and shoes, he refuses to change them. He says that the colour of your socks is not important in life. I disagree.

He thinks a fib is not a lie.

He fills our cupboards with things he never uses and won't ever let me throw them away. When I ask him how many cables one man needs, he says a lot.

I say he's stubborn. He says he's determined.

These are some of the things that make Peter cross about me:

Whenever we go to a restaurant I never want to sit at the first table that's offered. Sometimes I'm not even happy with the second.

I often wear the wrong clothes for the weather, which means that when it's cold I have to borrow his jacket.

I never carry tissues.

I pile the sink high with dirty dishes. Peter says this makes more work, as you have to take them out again to do the washing-up. I say it keeps things temporarily tidy.

I make him climb hills. He hates hills. And stairs.

He says I'm stubborn. I say I'm determined.

I sometimes wonder what would happen if we had children. Would we still argue or would there be other things to think about? Maybe it's because we don't have children that we argue as much as we do. Maybe we channel our pain through the small things. It's another aspect of our infertility that is unexplained.

The Infertility Diaries Part X

Something's happened to me. When I was a teenager, I was great with young children. I had a monopoly on babysitting in my neighbourhood and was in high demand. Now, all of a sudden, I feel self-conscious around them. Whenever I visit friends and family with babies I never ask to pick them up and, as if sensing my unease, they never offer. I have this paranoia that they think I might burst into tears or run off with them because I haven't got one of my own. I don't want to risk any embarrassment. In fact, I've started to notice that everyone is feeling more and more uncomfortable even mentioning babies around me. I know it's because they don't want to hurt my feelings but it actually makes things worse. They worry about telling me when someone gets pregnant because it will highlight that I'm not, and they've stopped inviting me to things where there will be children because they assume I won't enjoy it. Of course they're right. It does hurt. It hurts a lot. But, on balance, that's probably better than feeling like a leper.

SHIT HAPPENS

I am standing naked in front of the full-length mirror in our bedroom. It is now several months since my ectopic pregnancy and I still have three scars clearly visible across my tummy. One over my right fallopian tube, where they looked for the foetus first; one over my left tube, where they looked next; and one above my abdomen, where they eventually found it. It's strange to think that these scars will always be with me. A constant reminder of the journey my body has been on and the pregnancy that was there and then taken away. I can't help wondering if it's the closest I will ever get; whether, at the end of my life, these three small scars will be all I have to show that I was a mother.

My relationship with Peter has become increasingly strained over the last few months. We are struggling financially and emotionally to hold everything together. I know he feels that at times I'm pushing him away. Maybe I am.

We still have two embryos from our last round of IVF in the freezer at the clinic. We've been waiting for my body to recuperate fully before putting them back. But the time has come.

I know from my first frozen cycle that the process is relatively straightforward. It doesn't involve as many drugs; there's no operation under general anaesthetic; and to some extent a level of anxiety has been taken away because we already know that we have some embryos to put back. Traditionally a frozen embryo transfer has been considered marginally less likely to be successful than a fresh embryo transfer. However, some doctors now believe that if an embryo survives the thawing process it's likely to be of good quality and the chances of successful implantation are very high. I have been on the down-regulation drugs and am due at the clinic tomorrow for a blood test and scan to make sure that everything is going to plan and that they can start preparing my body to receive the embryos.

That night, Peter and I have one of the worst rows of our entire relationship. He has been out all day with some old friends he hasn't seen for ages and comes home smelling of drink. On any other day I might have made him some tea and toast and insisted on hearing the minutiae of proceedings. But today it is the red rag to the bull that has been lurking in the corner of my life for the last few months. I am furious at him for getting drunk. I am furious at him for spending money that we don't have. I am furious at him for lying – or so I believe – about how much he's drunk and how much money he's spent.

I start to shout. Then I start to throw things, picking up random objects from around the room and hurling them at him. Peter is sitting on the sofa, his hands over his head, trying to protect himself against the onslaught. I grab a bottle of unopened wine from the kitchen table. I unscrew it and pour it all over his head. He gets up and slips on the wet floorboards. As he lies there, covered in red wine, I start to kick him.

We sleep in separate rooms. Peter spends the night on the floor in his study in the attic. At five in the morning I go upstairs. He looks terrible. We both look terrible. Our eyes bloodshot with tiredness; our faces swollen from crying.

'I'm not going to go through with it,' I say quietly.

'Why not?'

'How can I contemplate even trying to bring a child into such a volatile relationship?'

'It's only volatile because of the drugs, the disappointment, everything we're going through. We love each other.'

'Do we? I don't know any more. Besides, it won't work anyway. What's the point? It never works.'

We are both silent for a few minutes. I fiddle with the tin of pens on Peter's desk.

'Listen,' he says softly. 'Let me take you to the clinic this morning. It doesn't mean you have to go through with it. Just keep the process moving for now; buy yourself some more time to think about it.'

It's a big thing for me to concede, but I do.

After we've been to the clinic Peter goes away for a few days, leaving me some space to think things over. We're both shocked by the ferocity of feeling that our row seems to have uncovered. To an outsider the subject of the argument might seem trivial, belying the anger that it invoked, but, as in so many faltering relationships, it's not always the things you argue about that are important. The truth is neither of us ever imagined we would be on this gruelling treadmill of medical probing, spiralling debt and continuing disappointment. Who would? We just fell in love, turned our own and others' lives upside down to be together, and then found ourselves on it. Now neither of us knows when or how to get off.

After a couple of days we speak on the phone.

'How are you feeling?' he asks.

'I still feel so angry with you,' I say.

'But all I did was have a few drinks.'

'That's one way of looking at it. Your way. It feels to me like you let me down. After everything we've been through, why would you risk jeopardising the process we're about to go through again by doing anything that would risk upsetting me?'

'You're making yourself upset. It's only jeopardised if you let it be.'

'Maybe. I'm not sure I've got the ability to be rational about this any more.'

'So what do you want to do?'

'I don't know,' I say. 'It's terrible timing, but I don't think I can give up on our embryos.'

'Me neither.'

There's a moment's silence before I continue.

'Well, there is one thing that I have been thinking about,' I say. 'But I'll only go through with it if you give me your permission.'

'You've got it,' he says immediately. And then, as an afterthought: 'Why? What is it?'

'I've been thinking that maybe I should go through the transfer without you. On my own. If it's successful – which it probably won't be – then we'll try and work things out.'

'And if it isn't?'

'Then I think we should separate.'

Just to be clear, I don't advocate this as a way of going through fertility treatment. It should be a time of hope and togetherness, not anger and separation. But life happens. Shit happens. Infertility happens.

There's another week or so to wait before my embryo transfer. Now that I have down-regulated, I am taking drugs to build up the lining of my womb so that it is at the optimum thickness for the embryos to implant. Peter is staying at his parents' house in the country while they are away.

We don't speak.

The day before the embryos are due back he sends me a text asking whether I want him to come for the transfer. I am surprised and confused that he knows when my appointment is, as it was only confirmed a couple of days ago. I immediately pick up the phone.

'Hello.'

'How are you?'

'Not great.'

'Me neither.'

'I just got your text. How do you know the embryos are going back tomorrow?' I ask.

'You told me, didn't you?' he says. Sheepishly.

'*No*. I only found out myself a couple of days ago. We haven't spoken, remember?'

'OK,' he says. 'I rang the clinic.'

'You did?'

'They didn't want to tell me at first. I think they thought it was a bit weird. But I said I'd double booked myself and was trying to sort things out so eventually they relented.'

I am touched by his deceptive determination.

'So, do you want me to come?' he asks.

'I'm not sure. I don't think so. I think I still want do it on my own.'

'OK. But I've got to come to Oxford tomorrow morning anyway for a dentist's appointment. I'll wait around until lunchtime. If you change your mind, call me.'

'I won't change my mind.'

It is easy to see in retrospect how the intractable positions we get ourselves into when we're angry just end up causing us more pain. At this moment I feel like I am protecting myself. I am ashamed to admit I don't care what Peter is feeling.

The following morning I dial Peter's mobile. It rings. Too many times. When he finally picks up I already know that it's too late.

'You didn't come, did you?'

'No,' he says. 'I felt so sad after we spoke. I cancelled my appointment.'

'But I've changed my mind.'

'What?' he says, surprised.

'I've changed my mind. I'm still upset with you but I was wrong. You should be here. Just in case.'

'Why didn't you ring me before?'

'I don't know.'

'I'll come now,' he says, hurriedly.

'You'll never get here in time.'

'I'm on my way. I'll meet you at the clinic.'

My appointment is at noon. The clinic is unusually quiet. I sit in the waiting room, flicking through a magazine. At twelve on the dot a nurse comes through.

'Are you ready?' she says brightly.

'Would you mind if we wait a few more minutes? My partner is on his way. He's running late but he's almost here.'

'OK,' she says. 'As it's quiet.'

Five minutes later she comes back.

'Is he here yet?'

'No,' I say. 'But don't worry, I can't keep you waiting any longer. Let's just make a start.'

'Is he in a red car by any chance?'

'Yes. Why?'

'I've just seen him swing into the car park at breakneck speed. I wondered whether that might be him.'

At the same moment the door swings open and Peter rushes in. We look at each other, then he pulls me towards him and kisses me.

'No time for that now,' the nurse says briskly. 'Save it until afterwards.'

If only she knew.

We are taken through to one of the consultation rooms and as the embryologist and nurse conduct the transfer it is as if nothing has happened. We are our usual laughing, loving selves. But afterwards, back in the car, memories of last week's events return and the atmosphere is brittle and uncertain. Peter drives me to the station so I can take the train to work. He pulls up on a double yellow line.

'Thanks for coming,' I say.

'Thank you for letting me.'

'So…' I pause for a moment. As I do, a bus comes up behind us and beeps its horn to move us along.

'So…?' Peter asks.

The bus beeps its horn again.

'So…I guess I'll call you when I know the result,' I say.

He nods. 'If that's what you want.'

And so a pause and the beep of a bus seal it. I get out of the car. Shut the door. And don't look back.

Sunday 21 March. The night of the annual Olivier Awards, the British theatre industry's equivalent of the Oscars. Everyone who is anyone in London theatre will be there, and one of our productions is up for several awards.

I have booked into a hotel for the night so I don't have to commute back to Oxford. When I arrive I'm told that I've been upgraded to a suite. I can't help wishing Peter were with me so that we could jump on the bed with excitement. But we haven't seen or spoken to each other for two weeks. I open my case and take out my dress and shoes. Then I take out a small paper bag containing the pregnancy test I have been given by the clinic. I lay it carefully next to the sink in the bathroom (which is bigger than our bedroom back home). Tomorrow is OTD. Official Test Day.

I go back into the bedroom, get dressed and then call a black cab to the Grosvenor Hotel. It's a good night: our production wins three awards. Everyone is ecstatic, especially as we are not expecting it. But at the end of the ceremony, as bottles of champagne are being lined up along the bar, I slip away from the celebrations. There's nothing as tedious as watching other people getting really drunk when you have to stay sober. I've started to get used to this over the last few years and, sadly, it's never been for a good reason. Maybe today will be different.

Back at the hotel, I get into bed. I feel strangely calm. Something does seem different this time. Usually I would be spotting by now. Perhaps even bleeding. But so far there has been nothing. I sleep deeply, wake up refreshed, and pad into the bathroom to take the test. The result is faint at first but slowly two lines start to appear, indicating that it's positive…POSITIVE!!!

Alone in the luxurious surroundings of my penthouse suite, it is almost as if I've stepped into someone else's glamorous life. I imagine I'm a movie star, thinking back on an awards ceremony where I had that one-night stand with the older, married director of my latest film. Now I've found out I'm pregnant by him. This can't actually be happening. Not to me. It's not how my life is.

But it *is* me, it *is* my life, and although I know this should be a joyous moment all I can think of is that I'm here alone, without Peter. I pick up the phone and call him. I feel lighter just hearing his voice, and his excitement when I tell him the news. Then I ring the clinic. It sounds strange listening to myself saying that I've done my pregnancy test and that it's positive, and then to hear their congratulations. They tell me that the next step is to come in for a scan in a few weeks' time. Apparently this is the earliest they will be able to see anything.

Over the next few days Peter and I talk on the phone a lot. He's still at his parents' house and we're both still tentative about the pregnancy and our relationship. Given all that has happened we both agree that it would be wrong to rush into things, so we decide that Peter will come down for my scan and we'll take it from there.

The following weekend I have arranged to meet up with Beth. I know she will be overjoyed for me and I have decided to save the news until I see her. We have a lovely girly lunch at the restaurant in the basement of Tate Britain and then visit the new Henry Moore exhibition. When I tell her the news she is so happy and excited, as I knew she would be. But over lunch I also have to tell her that earlier that same morning, nearly a week after my positive test, there has been a worrying sign. A smidgen of salmon pink. And we both know that a sign is a sign even when it's a smidgen.

The Infertility Diaries Part XI

Apparently you're supposed to focus on your womb: think positive thoughts; imagine everything is progressing well. That's what Zita West, the UK's holistic baby-making guru, says. Trouble is, I don't trust my tummy. I can't believe there's any woman who has lived with infertility that does.

THE FOOL

A few weeks ago I had dinner with a friend. She's one of the cleverest people I know (a double first from Oxford kind of clever). Over pudding she confided to me that she had recently been to see a psychic tarot-card reader who had been utterly amazing (her words). At the time I couldn't stop laughing and teasing her about when she was going to meet that tall dark handsome stranger. A few weeks later, I pick up the phone and book myself an appointment. Every rational bone in my body is screaming WHAT THE HELL ARE YOU DOING? But I still do it. Suddenly it isn't such a mad idea after all. In fact it might be my only hope of sanity.

I guess the moral of that story is: Be Careful What You Laugh At.

The tarot reader practises at a little shop in Covent Garden which is an Aladdin's cave of new age paraphernalia. As well as tarot they also offer reiki, psychic healing and aura readings. I take a seat in the waiting area upstairs, expecting a gothic Mystic Meg-type figure with staring eyes. It is quite a surprise when a big bubbly black woman named Barbara comes through and calls my name.

'Hello, my love,' she says. 'Have I read your cards before?'

'No. No one has.'

'All right then, let's see what we've got for you today.'

She asks me to cut the pack and lays several of them out on the table between us.

'Now here we have the Fool,' she says. 'That indicates a time of change.' She looks at me. 'Would that be right, my love?'

'Maybe,' I say.

'And next to that is the Lovers. I'm feeling that you might be on the cusp of a new relationship. Is that right?'

'No. I don't think so.'

'All right, so let's see then,' she says. 'Well, we also have the Tower, which is associated with decision. And alongside that is the Emperor, which is associated with power. Maybe you're considering a change of career? Or some other sort of life change?'

'Erm, maybe.'

She carries on in this vein for a while, with me giving monosyllabic answers to each of her questions. I am determined not to give too much away so that I can be certain I'm not influencing anything she says. So far there has been nothing decisive.

Eventually she stops looking at the cards and turns towards me.

'Listen, my love, you're going to have give me more to work with here. Is there something specific you want to know?'

'Yes.'

'Well, what is it?'

'I don't want to say. I want you to tell me.'

'It doesn't really work like that, my love. Maybe if you could give me an indication then we can see what the cards say.'

'OK,' I say a little reluctantly. 'I want to know about my pregnancy.'

'Your pregnancy? Why? Are you pregnant?'

'Yes.'

'Right,' she says slowly. 'So what do you want to know exactly?'

'I want to know what's going to happen.'

'What's going to happen? I'm not sure I understand.'

This isn't how I envisaged things would go but

I've started now so I might as well explain.

'I've been trying to conceive for a long time,' I say. 'I've been through a lot of fertility treatment. I want to know whether this time it's finally going to work.'

'Ah, I see, you want to know whether you're going to have a miscarriage?'

'Yes.'

Throughout this exchange she has been looking at the cards, tapping each of them with her long fingernails. The moment I answer in the affirmative she puts down the pack and looks at me.

'And why do you think you might have a miscarriage?'

'I don't know; just my luck, I guess. I suppose I've come here because I want to know whether it's finally going to change.'

'You're not spotting, are you?' she asks (a little flippantly).

'Actually, yes.'

'Now listen to me, my love, spotting doesn't mean anything. Lots of women spot and have perfectly normal pregnancies. Stop worrying. I'm sure things will be fine.'

I look at her and don't reply. It's all very well, I think, but I'm not lots of women.

Then she turns to the cards again and finishes the reading. She focuses on the ones that herald positive change, which seem to be most of them in some way or another. I leave the shop none the wiser.

I never told anyone about that afternoon. Not my friend who recommended her. Not even Peter. Sometimes you want to believe that someone somewhere can tell you what the future holds. The truth is nobody can. Although I guess you could say the Fool card was right – I definitely felt one.

The Infertility Diaries Part XII

I went into Waterstone's today and allowed myself to look at baby books for the first time. I even decided to buy one. It's got fabulous pictures showing how your foetus is developing on a day-by-day basis. But as I stood at the counter, book in hand, I couldn't help feeling like a fraud. What if I'm wasting my money? What if I never get past the first few pages? What if the book ends up gathering dust on the shelf, waiting for me to take it to Oxfam for someone who can really use it?

MINI-MOLLY

A few days later I wake up in the middle of the night. There is a slow, dull ache across my lower back and I can feel blood between my legs. I know that if I ring the clinic they will tell me the usual: don't worry, it might not mean the worst. But I am thinking the worst, so as soon as it's morning I call a taxi to take me to the clinic.

The receptionist looks at me with shocked surprise when I tell her that I haven't got an appointment but I think I'm miscarrying and want to see someone. She calls a nurse, who looks at me with shocked disapproval.

'You shouldn't just come into the clinic like this,' she scolds. 'You should have called us first.'

'I'm sorry,' I lie. I'm not sorry. I know what would have happened if I'd rung. Right now, I need more than that.

'OK, as you're here I'll give you a scan,' the nurse says reluctantly. 'But I have to tell you, it's very unlikely we'll be able to see anything. It's far too early.'

She takes me into a consultation room and tells me to get undressed.

'Well, I can see a pregnancy sac, which is a good sign,' she says within a few minutes. 'It's possible that both embryos implanted and you've lost one, which has caused this bleeding. The good news is there is definitely still one sac, but it really is too early to see anything else. You will need to come back on your official scan day.'

'Thank you so much,' I say gratefully as I climb off the trolley and put my trousers back on.

'It's all right,' she replies. 'But don't come in like that again. Ring us next time.'

As I leave the clinic I don't know whether to feel happy that I still seem to be pregnant or sad that I might have just lost a twin. Mostly I feel happy.

As soon as I get into work, I switch on my computer and email Peter:

Come home.

A minute later his reply pops into my inbox:

Are you sure?

I email back:

Never been surer.

When I get off the train that evening, he's waiting for me outside the station. He wraps his arms around me.

'I've brought the car,' he says. 'I'm going to make sure you take things easy from now on.'

'Easy? I'm not sure I know the meaning of that word.'

'Well you might as well make the most of it, because if our baby is anything like you, as soon as it's born you're never going to have it easy again.'

'And if it's anything like you, it will be asking for rum in its milk by the time it's six months.'

'The kid's got taste!' he says.

We both laugh.

The week-and-a-half wait until the day of my official scan is agony. When it finally arrives I give the nurse a hurried explanation of the events since my positive test. Just so that she knows I am not assuming everything is going to be fine. Just to make it easier for her if it isn't.

As I lie on the trolley she stares at the screen intently, doing something that makes a repetitive clicking sound. After forever she turns towards us.

'I'm sorry for the wait,' she says. 'I wanted to be sure.'

We look at her uncertainly.

'Well,' she says, 'the good news is that I can confirm you are pregnant and I can see a strong foetal heartbeat, which is a very encouraging sign.'

'And the bad news?' I ask immediately, convinced that there's never one without the other these days.

'Yes, I'm afraid there is something that's not quite so good,' she replies. 'The foetus seems to be about half the size it should be by this stage.'

The clicking sound had been her measuring it. She turns the screen towards us so we can see for ourselves. Peter and I look at each other and then at the tiny fluttering spot, fighting for its life.

'So what happens next?' I ask.

'We will need to book you in for another scan in a couple of weeks' time. We will know more then. In the meantime, if you get any more heavy bleeding

I suggest you go straight to the Early Pregnancy Unit at the John Radcliffe.'

Over the next few days Peter does a lot of talking to my tummy. For years now we have dreamt of having a little girl called Molly. It's the only name we both agree on. So we name her 'Mini-Molly', and with all our hope we will for her to keep growing. But the bleeding continues and within a few days is pretty heavy, so we decide to go to the hospital.

After years of experiencing the weirdness of infertility clinics, it now feels even weirder to be in a place where regular pregnant people go. We are surrounded by other parents-to-be, waiting for their first three-month scan. As we don't have an appointment we have to wait to be seen as an emergency. After three nerve-wracking hours we are finally called into the scanning room, where there are two nurses – one who scans, the other who enters the details into a computer. I am immediately struck by how bright and breezy they both seem. They're not like infertility nurses, hardened by disappointment. These nurses are clearly used to the joy of showing a couple the new life they have created on screen for the first time.

They ask me my name, address, how many weeks pregnant I am. I feel like saying that they are wasting their time going through the usual rigmarole. They might as well do the scan, confirm the worst, and save the space on the database. But I go with it; we're only minutes away anyhow.

The scanning nurse conducts the ultrasound through my stomach. I've never experienced this before, but I've seen it so many times on film and TV that it feels familiar. I allow myself to dream for a moment that I'm a normal person attending a routine antenatal appointment. The nurse massages the cold gel into my stomach as she moves the probe around, trying to get a good view of my uterus.

'There it is,' she says suddenly.

'Pardon?' I reply.

'Your little jelly bean – strong foetal heartbeat, now let's just measure it.'

'What? Really?' I say, confused.

'Yes, really,' she says. 'Everything seems absolutely fine.'

She calls out the measurements to the other nurse sitting at the computer. Not only is Mini-Molly's heartbeat still strong, but she has grown to 9 millimetres and has almost doubled in size since our first scan. I steal a glance at Peter, seeing the relief and happiness on his face.

We leave the hospital elated. They even give us a photo. One of those grainy black and white images with a little dot which means nothing to anyone except its mum and dad. All that talking to my tummy worked. Things are going be fine.

Another week passes and eventually the day for our follow-up scan at the clinic arrives. As we sit in the waiting room, I notice Peter tearing off a scrap of paper from his notebook and writing something on it.

'What are you doing?' I ask.

'I'll tell you later,' he says cryptically.

Generally I wouldn't (couldn't) leave that hanging, but today I have bigger things on my mind. I am nervous about the scan. Although I'm nearly eight weeks pregnant, I know there is a long way to go before we're through and out the other side.

The same nurse who scanned us the first time collects us from the waiting area.

'How are you both doing?' she asks.

'OK,' I reply. 'I've still been bleeding on and off. We took your advice and went to the Early Pregnancy Unit. They did a scan and said everything was looking fine but I'm still anxious.'

'Of course,' she says. 'I understand.'

She stares at the screen intently, making those clicking noises again. She's measuring it. That must be a good sign. None of us speaks until she finally stops and turns.

'Jessica, Peter, I'm afraid there's no easy way of

saying this but the foetal heartbeat seems to have stopped.'

'But how?' I demand. 'At the hospital they told us the heartbeat was really strong. They said the foetus had doubled in size.'

'Yes, it has grown since I last saw you but I definitely can't see a heartbeat. I'm really sorry.'

'What does that mean? What can we do?'

'Sadly there isn't anything. I'm afraid it means that you're going to miscarry.'

I look away and take a deep breath to try and compose myself. Then I turn back to her.

'So when will it happen?' I ask.

'It's difficult to be sure exactly. A week. Maybe two. We could do what is called a D & C and remove the embryo under general anaesthetic, but we much prefer to let things happen naturally. I'm so sorry, I know this must be hard for you.'

'It's all right,' I say quietly. 'I'm used to hard.'

On the way home in the car our silence is heavy. Then I remember the slip of paper. Peter admits that he had been so sure everything would be fine that he'd written down that he thought Mini-Molly would be 16 millimetres today, so he could impress me with his mathematical prowess later. I love him so much for his optimism, in spite of its futility.

We get home and sit down on the sofa in the

front room. The thought of spending the next few weeks with our baby dead inside me is heartbreaking. Neither of us knows what to say. Eventually Peter gets up.

'Shall I make a cup of tea?' he asks.

'OK,' I reply.

Sometimes there is nothing more you can say. Or do.

The Infertility Diaries Part XIII

Molly will be fair and long-limbed. There's nothing you can do about genetics. I have this image of us as a family holidaying in the South of France. She is about eight. We watch as she runs fearlessly towards the hotel swimming pool, dives in and swims like a fish to the other end. Hopping out of the pool she wraps herself in a big towel and curls up on a sun-lounger with a book. She reads voraciously, disdaining her tablet for words on a page. That's our girl.

I can't helping thinking that the nurse might have made a mistake. Maybe Mini-Molly's heart is still beating and she just didn't see it. Maybe the miscarriage will never come. It has happened. Google it and you'll see.

JERUSALEM

I have this theory – not statistically proven, I hasten to add – that every theatre creates one production each decade that defines it. For the Donmar Warehouse in the 1990s it was *The Blue Room* with Nicole Kidman and Iain Glen. For the National Theatre in the 2000s it would have to be *War Horse*. I'd lay money on it being Jez Butterworth's *Jerusalem* for the Royal Court in the 2010s (even though we haven't got to the end of them yet).

I missed the show when it first opened – this was less to do with not being able to get a ticket, and more to do with the fact that I couldn't face the thought of sitting through three hours of theatre. Believe me, there isn't anyone who works in theatre who doesn't ask what the running time is when walking into an auditorium, then breathe a silent sigh of relief when they're told that it's going to be one and a half hours straight through without an interval. You don't choose to go to a three-hour play unless you have to, or it's unmissable. It soon became clear that *Jerusalem,* and particularly Mark Rylance's tour de force performance as Rooster, was the latter.

After its run at the Royal Court the show

transferred to the West End, and I managed to get a couple of tickets for the final Saturday matinee. It was a sunny day and the atmosphere outside the theatre was more like a rock concert than a theatre performance. There were touts offering tickets at ludicrous prices, and I overheard an American woman saying how delighted she was to have won hers in a bidding war on eBay. It always astonishes and delights me when a theatre production generates this much interest. Perhaps that's the reaction of someone who knows only too well how difficult it can be to give away tickets for nothing when you've made a show that no one wants to come and see.

I was seeing the play with an old friend of mine from university called Ella who was running late. She was coming direct from an Internet-instigated blind date, which she often does on weekend lunchtimes because she says there's less pressure and you can always find a good excuse to get away quickly if you need to. They were ringing the one-minute call bell when she arrived and we hurried to our seats in the stalls. The sense of anticipation in the auditorium was palpable. There was no time to catch up before the lights went down and the play began.

In the interval there was the customary queue for the ladies' toilets – proof if ever it were needed that all Victorian theatre architects were men. My tactic (which I offer as an insider's recommendation to everyone) is to hang on until just a few minutes before the show is about to restart. Invariably the queue is down to only two or three by then and you've always got more time than the front of house staff want you to think you have.

I closed the cubicle door, undid my trousers, and as I bent down there was a massive rush of blood.

Nothing can prepare you for the shock of a miscarriage – even when you're expecting it. It's often said that they are extremely common, and some women who miscarry don't even know that they have conceived as it can be little more than a heavy period. But I have been having periods for twenty-five years and this felt nothing like it. Apart from the enormous amount of blood, it was thick and globular. Even a Tampax Super Plus wouldn't have stood a chance for more than a couple of minutes. But I should be so lucky. I didn't have anything with me at all, which you can read as either stupidity or denial.

I realise that most people in this situation would probably have left the theatre. This would probably be the sensible thing to do. But my friend Ella was in the auditorium and I could hear the furious ringing of the call bell. The show was now really about to re-start. So I created a makeshift sanitary towel with a wodge of toilet paper (show me a woman who has never done that), tied my jumper round my waist to hide the blood, and went back to my seat.

I must have gone very pale because Ella looked concerned.

'Are you all right?' she asked.

'I'm not quite sure how to say this,' I whispered, 'but I'm having a miscarriage.'

'Oh my god, shall we leave?' she said.

'It's OK, I was expecting it but it's a bit of a shock nonetheless. I'll explain afterwards.'

And with that the lights went down on the second half.

When I look back at all the plays I've seen in my life there are only a few that really stand out. *Jerusalem* will always be one of them. I feel lucky to be able to say that I saw the original production, with the performance that has earned Rylance a god-like status among actors. But as the audience rose to its feet at the end of the play to give the cast a standing ovation, all I could feel was blood running down my leg. Sadly that's the thing that I will most and always remember.

The Infertility Diaries Part XIV

*In my darker moments (of which these days there are many)
I wonder whether my infertility is some sort of punishment
for how Peter and I got together. For the pain we caused to
others. Maybe I don't deserve to be a mother. Maybe this is
my retribution.*

ANGER MANAGEMENT

After the miscarriage we go to see our consultant.
He is as sympathetic as ever but I am getting sick of
sympathy; I just want some answers.

'I don't understand what's happening,' I say. 'I've
now been through this process six times. I've had
two biochemical pregnancies, one ectopic, now a
miscarriage. What am I not doing right?'

'Nothing,' he says. 'I know it might not seem like
it, but these are all very good indications that you
will get pregnant. If you were a machine, I would
simply say keep going and sooner or later it will
work. But I realise you're not a machine; there's an
emotional and financial cost to all this as well.'

'But there must be a reason I can't seem to
sustain a pregnancy,' I say.

I steal a glance at Peter, remembering our many

conversations in which I have denied the existence of stress.

'Do you think it could be stress?' I ask.

'Unlikely,' he says going into lecture mode. 'All the studies that have been done indicate that stress is not a significant factor. If you look at conception rates of women living in poor or war-torn countries they are no lower than those for Western women. There was also a seminal study done on women who had been raped, which found that pregnancy rates amongst them were no different than for women who had conceived in a loving relationship.'

'Well what about my immune system? I've recently read about these things called natural killer cells that attack the foetus. Do you think that could be it?'

'The doctor who pioneered this theory was based in California – he's dead now – and there are a small number of doctors in the UK who practise his methodology, but there have been absolutely no clinical trials to prove its efficacy. Whilst I wouldn't say that these treatments would harm you, there are no grounds to suggest they would make any difference at all.'

'With respect, there must be a reason. Maybe science doesn't know what it is yet. Maybe they won't find it out in my lifetime. But there will be a reason.'

'Possibly.'

'Well, go on, hazard a guess. What do you think

is wrong with me? I won't hold you to it, but in your professional judgement, what the hell is going on?'

He pauses. 'Jessica, I don't know. All I can say is that you are either very unusual, or *very* unlucky.'

We say goodbye and as the door closes behind us I look at Peter.

'You were a bit hard on him,' he says.

'Was I?'

'Well, you used the phrase, "With respect". It's always a giveaway.'

'Well, with respect, there *must* be a reason.'

'Perhaps. But it's not his fault. He's trying to do his best for us.'

'Is he? I'm fed up with being told that all the indications are that if we keep on trying I will get pregnant. It just means we do what we did last time and then we don't.'

'This clinic has got us further than any other. They deserve another chance.'

'Maybe.'

'And maybe, in the meantime, you need to do something about your anger.'

'Angry? Me?'

'Yes. You.'

Peter probably has a point. My anger is becoming more and more of a problem. With us; with our doctor; with everybody. And so a month after my miscarriage I find myself in East Grinstead on a Friday morning. My work colleagues think I'm away for a long weekend, which, strictly speaking, I am. But there isn't a hotel with a spa in sight. Instead, I've booked myself on to an intensive weekend of Anger Management.

When I arrive two women are already there having coffee. I help myself to a cup and join them in polite conversation. One of them is the programme administrator, the other a Scottish woman who is attending the course that weekend. The first thing the administrator says to me is that there have been a number of dropouts, so there will now be only three of us taking part. This isn't good news as it means there will be nowhere to hide. A few minutes later a man, probably late twenties, comes in: the last of our trio. He seems very nervous, which instantly makes me feel more relaxed.

Then the course tutor arrives. A small, round South African who bounces with self-assurance.

'Hi,' he says, shaking my hand. 'I'm Mike.'

'Jessica,' I say.

He looks me up and down.

'Are you pregnant?' he asks.

'Pardon?'

'Are you pregnant?'

'No.'

'Mike, you can't say things like that,' the administrator hisses.

'Sorry,' he says.

'You probably will be later,' I say (quietly).

I look down at myself surreptitiously. I am wearing a long baggy grey jumper over skinny jeans and boots. I thought I looked casually sophisticated. But clearly the outfit also makes me look fat. Or pregnant. Maybe I am fat, because I'm definitely not pregnant.

Let's just say this isn't a good start to the weekend. I'm hurt (what woman wouldn't be?), and I'm also angry that the tutor of the course could be so tactless. I guess I'm in the right place to deal with it, but at this precise moment I feel too angry to think about trying. All morning I continue to fume, distancing myself from the group by giving brief and cautious answers.

At lunch Mike turns to me and says, 'Jessica, can I guess what you do for a living?'

'OK,' I say suspiciously.

'Are you a recruitment consultant?'

'No.'

I look at him intently, waiting for the next question. It doesn't come so I don't volunteer the right answer either. I think you could say this isn't going well.

In the afternoon session Mike leads us into a more in-depth discussion about why each of us has come on the course. The man in his twenties describes an incident he was involved in a few weeks ago. He had been at a pub with some friends in his home town when a guy standing next to him at the bar said something – he couldn't even remember what it was – and he found himself turning round and hitting him in the face. He has no idea why he did it, and he is shaking so much as he tells the story, it is clear that this is the truth.

The Scottish woman says that she and her husband have terrible rows and she's worried about the effect it's having on their children. She is explosive. He is passive aggressive. They have both agreed to do the course separately to try to find techniques to deal with it.

Then it's my turn. I contemplate lying but then think of the four hundred quid I've shelled out to do the course. So I take a deep breath and tell the group that I'm angry with the hand that life has dealt me, and that recently I've felt this more than ever.

'And why's that?' Mike asks.

'Because after spending years trying to get pregnant, I finally did, and then I had a miscarriage.'

For the first time that day Mike is silent.

That'll teach him.

By the end of the day I am starting to feel better. When I get back to the hotel I am staying at for the weekend, I crack open a bottle of sparkling water from the minibar – the course has a no-alcohol rule – and contemplate what I've learned. I think the most salient lesson is that being angry with other people ultimately only hurts you. I guess my own feelings that day have proved the theory.

The rest of the weekend is more enjoyable. We learn Mike's eight steps to managing your anger and we get to know each other's relationships with anger intimately. Given that we all spend most of our lives with the same people, having more or less the same conversations, there is something special about developing a deep and honest connection with a group of strangers over the course of a weekend. At times it starts to feel like we are in intensive group therapy. Mike, in his now familiar blunt manner, makes acute and sometimes painful observations about each one of us. It feels like every aspect of our lives, not just our anger, is under the microscope.

By the end of the course I think the most important insight I've had is that anger is just the reaction to something else – something deeper going on inside. You have to start by working out what that is before you can overcome it. It makes me realise that I'm not really an angry person at all. It's just a by-product of how sad and disappointed

I am that my life isn't working out as I planned.

And the hard thing? I still have absolutely no idea what to do about it.

The Infertility Diaries Part XV

I guess I have to admit that Mike had a point. When I reached my mid-thirties I started to notice what I can only describe as a small rubber ring developing round my tummy, like I'm wearing one of those all-in-one swimming costumes for toddlers with a float stitched in. I keep thinking I must do something about it. A hundred sit-ups each morning, something like that. Then I think, what's the point if I'm going to get pregnant? Much better to wait until afterwards and then really attack it. But I've been saying that for years now. The excuse is starting to wear a little thin.

THE STONEMASONS ARMS

I'll always remember today. One of my best members of staff handed in his notice. It's a right pain when that happens. I feel like bursting into tears and accusing him of desertion, but I've learnt the hard way that there is no point in getting upset and taking it personally. So I throw my arms round him, say congratulations, and start working out what the hell to do next. But I digress. It's neither his resignation nor my noble response for which the day will be remembered.

After work I take him out for a drink with a couple of other colleagues to celebrate his new job. Spontaneous nights out are always the best. A couple of bottles of wine in and we are having a brilliant time plotting our takeover of the National Theatre. Then, all of a sudden, my head starts pounding and the room starts to swirl. I lay forward on the table and say: 'I'm sorry, I suddenly feel really drunk.'

I can feel embarrassment looking down on me. This is hardly how the boss should behave. But I can't lift my head to do anything about it. I start to feel nauseous. That telltale sensation of saliva in the back of the throat.

'I'm sorry,' I say again. 'I think I'm going to be sick.'

Then I lift my head, swivel round in my chair, and throw up on the floor of the Stonemasons Arms.

My colleagues seem to be taking the situation in their stride. One of them immediately goes over to the bar to get a cloth; another moves my bag and coat away from the vomit. I lay my head helplessly back on the table.

'I need to go home,' I say.

'You can't go back to Oxford on your own like this,' one of them says. 'Why don't you come and stay with me?'

'I can't,' I say. 'I've got to go home.'

'Well let us ring Peter and get him to come and pick you up.'

'He's not there,' I say. 'He's away working.'

'Then why don't you stay with one of us? Or your parents? Or a friend?'

'I can't,' I say more forcefully. 'I *have* to go home.'

'But why?'

'I just have to.' And then, because I can't think of anything else to say, I tell the truth: 'I'm going through IVF. I have to go home to take my drugs.'

I sense a beat of silent surprise after my unexpected revelation. Whilst my ectopic pregnancy had become common knowledge, and a few senior staff also knew about my miscarriage, I had never explicitly told anyone that these had all been the result of IVF treatment.

'Can you call me a taxi?' I say.

'A taxi? To Oxford? That will cost a fortune. If you have to go home why don't you let one of us take you to Paddington and put you on the train.'

'No,' I say firmly. 'Call me a taxi. I don't care what it costs.'

I don't have another choice. I feel terrible –

almost on the verge of unconsciousness – but I am halfway through the stimulation phase of another round of IVF and I have to do whatever it takes to get home. A couple of hours later, fifty miles and one hundred and fifty quid down, I crawl into bed, give myself my injection, and fall asleep in relief.

The next day I feel so ashamed. Added to the embarrassment of disclosing we are going through IVF, I also feel utterly irresponsible. Why have I risked jeopardising yet another round of treatment and all the money it costs by going out and getting drunk?

The only explanation I can find is that for years I have persuaded myself that carrying on as normal and not telling anyone what I am going through is a good thing. But in doing so my infertility and IVF treatment has become such a routine and hidden part of my life that I haven't been making any allowances for how it might be affecting me on any level: from the effect that fertility drugs might have on a few glasses of wine in the pub; to the impact that years of unsuccessful treatment might be having on my psychological health.

Last night was a wake-up call, and as soon as my hangover is gone I start to listen.

The Infertility Diaries Part XVI

I bumped into a former work colleague yesterday. I hadn't seen him for about a year, and almost as soon as we started chatting he said, 'I've got some news: Celia and I are having a baby!' Everyone I see regularly these days is so tentative and tactful about making pregnancy announcements around me that his excited openness came as quite a surprise. In fact, it was so discombobulating that, for a moment, I actually responded with spontaneous enthusiasm myself. Just like a normal person.

THE POINT

Sunday, 21 November 2010. My fortieth birthday. I have invited my closest family and friends to a slap-up Sunday lunch at St John in Clerkenwell, one of my favourite restaurants. Just as pudding is coming to an end, I stand up and tinkle my glass with a spoon.

'First of all, I want to thank everyone for coming today and fulfilling my dream to have my forty favourite people at my fortieth birthday. It means so much to me to have you all here doing what I love doing best: eating!'

Everyone laughs.

'I've never been big on birthdays,' I continue, 'but I've decided that it is really important to mark and celebrate each decade of your life. The last ten years have been a wonderful time for me in many ways. I got to fulfil my childhood dream of running a theatre, and I met Peter, who has been a continuing source of joy – and frustration.'

I smile at Peter and everyone laughs again.

'However, as some of you are aware, the last decade has also been a really difficult one for us. We would love to have children but have struggled to get pregnant. We have been through a long and gruelling process of tests and treatment and there has been a lot of disappointment...'

I look around the room. Everyone is watching me intently.

'But,' I continue, 'I thought you might also all like to know that today, in addition to my fortieth birthday, we finally have something else to celebrate. I am three months pregnant. With twins!'

There is a spontaneous cheer and everyone gets up and rushes forward to hug us both.

It is a perfect moment. One that I have dreamed about. But our seventh round of IVF, which made this dream possible, has ended in another biochemical pregnancy and early miscarriage. Even more disheartening, it is my worst response to treatment so far. Five eggs collected. Three fertilised. Two embryos put back on Day 3. Spotting. Positive early pregnancy test (home kit, taken in desperation on Day 10 of the two-week wait) and then negative pregnancy test (clinic kit, taken on the official test date). Logically, I know that the incident in the Stonemasons Arms can't be the only reason it has failed again, but nevertheless I blame myself.

I wonder for a few days about whether to have the party still but it no longer feels like there is anything I want to mark or celebrate. The idea of standing up in front of anyone and saying anything is unbearable. So I ditch the idea, turn to my default position, and decide to spend the night of my fortieth birthday in a luxury hotel in the Adirondacks instead.

Now, I know what you're thinking. Why of all places the Adirondacks? Either that, or where the hell are they? And how can you afford it? Well, the week before my birthday I have to go to New York for work, so I decide to stay on there and Peter flies out to join me. The Adirondacks is a national park in the north of New York State, which I mistakenly thought wasn't far from Manhattan. But – just for future reference – whilst it is in New York State it is also a six-hour drive from the capital, and make that seven hours if you get lost and stopped for speeding. Both of which we did.

The other guests at the hotel are incredulous that we have driven all this way for just twenty-four hours. Everyone else is American and they clearly think it's a case of mad dogs and Englishmen. Frankly, though, we couldn't afford to stay for more than a night. One of my great weaknesses is expensive hotels, and this is definitely the most expensive night of my life. So far.

The hotel, which is perched on the side of a huge lake, originally belonged to the Rockefeller family and was their summer retreat from the city. It is so exclusive that it's not signposted and you have to follow instructions that include: *from the crossroads, check your odometer and after exactly 18.6 kilometers, turn left on to an unmarked road and continue to the end*.

When we arrive at the hotel gates they are closed and forbidding to strangers. We ring the bell and introduce ourselves over the intercom. As they slowly open, a man comes over to the car and says: 'Welcome to the Point.'

He directs us straight ahead to the main entrance. There, waiting for us, are two more members of staff. As we step out of the car one takes the keys and the other says: 'You're just in time for lunch. Would you like to start with a glass of champagne?'

Now *this* is my sort of hotel.

Although you may have to take out a second

mortgage to afford a room for the night at the Point, one small bonus is that, once you have, everything is included. You could drink champagne all day if you wanted to. And if you wanted oysters to accompany it you could probably have them too. Another thing about the hotel is that you have all your meals, except breakfast, at the same table as the other guests. It's rather like being at a posh country house party. Either that or a piece of site-specific theatre.

If truth be told we aren't *just in time for lunch*. We are late. The other guests are already sitting down and there are two empty chairs at the table. We are frazzled from the long drive, and were we more accustomed to such a milieu we might ask to freshen up or even take lunch in our room. But we're English. We're polite. We receive our glass of champagne gratefully and say we'd be more than happy to go straight to the table.

I introduce myself to the man sitting on my left. We start to chat. It turns out he's the ex-Chief of Staff to the Governor of New York. I can hardly contain my excitement. It's almost as if I'm sitting next to Leo from *The West Wing*. After lunch I compare notes with Peter, who is equally excited. He was sitting next to a man who told him he was a probate lawyer. When Peter said to him that he'd just been reading in *Vanity Fair* about an interesting probate case regarding an American billionairess, the man had said: 'Yes, that is an interesting case. In fact, it's one of mine.'

It's a wild and windy day. Most of the guests tell us they are planning to spend the afternoon relaxing by the open fires in their bedrooms. Peter gets a wistful look in his eyes. But I've got other plans. We're going out for a walk. As beautiful as the hotel is, it seems madness to come to one of America's most spectacular national parks and stay indoors. Besides, it's my birthday, so even if I already get my way most of the time, this time it is fully justified.

We set off on one of the designated trails around the estate. As the staff wave us off they say: 'Don't forget to stop at "Camp David". There will be something waiting for you.'

After about an hour we reach a single-storey log cabin in the middle of the woods (a small but perfectly formed copy of the country retreat of the President of the United States). The place is deserted but there's a fire crackling in the hearth and a flask of hot chocolate on the table with a bottle of Baileys standing next to it. Beside it a handwritten note: *Jessica and Peter. Just a little something to warm you up*.

Now *this* is my sort of walk (and Peter's too).

Dinner at the Point is a black-tie affair. That night there are ten guests: Peter and me; *West Wing* Leo and his wife; Mr Probate and his wife; a surgeon and his wife; and a young couple in their twenties – he is a foreign correspondent for *Time* magazine and later admits to reviewing hotels for them on the side, which all but confirms that they are on a lig (lucky things). It makes for an interesting evening and Peter does a brilliant job of keeping up with American dinner party conversation, which includes whether Barack Obama has made any impact in office and the pros and cons of gun ownership. He even does a good job of explaining the rules of cricket and cracking a few jokes about American versus English football. One of the things I love most about Peter is that he knows a little about most things and can talk to anyone about anything. In this respect he's totally unlike me, as these days I seem to have only three subjects I can talk about with confidence: work; being me; and (coming up on the inside) infertility.

As dinner draws to a close the hotel manager gets everyone's attention and says that there is just one more Point tradition we have to indulge in. In the days of the Rockefellers the evening would always end round the campfire by the lake, everyone toasting marshmallows and telling each other stories.

We all go back to our rooms to get changed into something warm. While we're there, I pop to the loo and get a bit of a shock to see that I appear to be bleeding a little.

'What's wrong?' Peter says as I emerge from the bathroom.

'Nothing, really.'

'That means something.'

'It's just I seem to be bleeding.'

'Is it your period?'

'No, that's what's confusing. My period finished last week. It's far too early for another.'

If I were younger, I wouldn't give it a second thought. I wouldn't even have mentioned it. But now, on the eve of my fortieth birthday, it seems to be unequivocal evidence of my advancing age and failing reproductive system. I lie down on the floor in front of the open fire in our beautiful bedroom in the Adirondacks and start to cry.

We never saw the bonfire or ate a marshmallow that night. Looking back it seems such a waste. However, I have since met several women who confessed that they too ended their fortieth birthday in tears. Everyone has their reasons, but if you haven't yet had a baby and want one, it's definitely the point you start to feel that the egg timer's on the final turn.

The Infertility Diaries Part XVII

I have recently become obsessed with listening to old episodes of Desert Island Discs *on BBC iPlayer. I am most drawn to interviews with women, looking to see something in them that I recognise in myself, I guess. Lately I've listened to a few with women who never had children: Debbie Harry, Tracey Emin, Cath Kidston, Janet Street-Porter. In spite of their professional success, their childlessness seems to have left something missing. I can't help wondering if it's going to be the same for me.*

IT'S DIFFERENT FOR BOYS

Like many people, I have always had a secret fantasy that one day I'll be invited to appear on *Desert Island Discs*. I've already picked out my eight tracks, and one of them will definitely be by Joe Jackson. Either *Is She Really Going Out with Him?* or *It's Different for Girls* – a reminder of the many hours I spent as a teenager lying on my bedroom floor, with my head to the speaker, thinking about my unrequited first love.

And let's face it, Joe Jackson was right: it *is* different for women. Men definitely drew the long straw when it comes to having children. The oldest father on record is in his nineties, and, for men, having children later in life is often a badge of celebrity or success. From Picasso to Michael Douglas, Charlie Chaplin to Rod Stewart. Unfortunately, God or evolution (you choose) has worked things out differently for women. By her forties, a woman's lifetime supply of eggs is fast diminishing and natural conception becomes much harder. When you read about women giving birth in their late forties and fifties, it is mainly because they have used donor eggs from a younger woman. At the moment, the only way to significantly increase the number of older women giving birth to their own biological children is for their eggs to be routinely frozen in their twenties and thirties for later use.

I can't help thinking how unfair the disparity is between men and women's fertility. It's now perfectly normal and natural for men to focus on their careers and avoid commitment until their forties and fifties. And why shouldn't they? As life expectancy increases there really is no need for them to settle down until they've exhausted all the fun and freedom that youth offers. But for women, the later we leave having children, the harder it is for us to conceive naturally. Add to this the still unknown effects of the high-flying, stressful careers that feminism has encouraged us to pursue in our twenties and thirties and the whole thing looks decidedly risky. This seems particularly ironic given that, on average, a woman's life expectancy is longer than a man's. But we are either going to need a major advance in medical science or a monumental shift in societal thinking for things to change anytime soon. Meanwhile, the fertility industry (or more precisely the infertility industry) is set to keep on growing.

Yet, just to prove that life is always fair in its unfairness, it's also true that whereas fertility favours men, the infertility industry is largely about women. Take the 'producing room', with its inbuilt assumption that men can basically masturbate under any conditions. Can you imagine if all the women going through fertility treatment had to go into these rooms and achieve an orgasm? There either wouldn't be as many babies born from IVF or something would have to be done to improve them. It may be true that women have to undergo the majority of tests and treatment, but essentially most of it's done to them. Men, on the other hand, have to go into that little room and actively produce the goods. It's a lot of pressure.

I think the lack of consideration for what men have to go through is one of the really hard and unspoken things about the infertility process. The social stigma surrounding a man who can't get a woman pregnant is still immensely strong. And many men's instinct, however wrong, is to blame themselves for their perceived inability to do what men should be able to do. But it's rarely discussed, and whilst women increasingly have places they can turn to for advice and support, men still don't. So, yes, Joe Jackson was right, it *is* different for girls. But where infertility's concerned there's no doubt that it's different, and difficult, for boys too.

HOPE YOU'RE HAPPY TOO

'Peter?'

'Yes.'

'I've realised I don't know what you feel.'

'About what?'

'About life.'

'That's a big question for six in the morning.'

'I've been thinking about it for a while.'

'I haven't.'

'Well think about it now.'

'OK. Life is a gift.'

'Even when you can't get what you want?'

'Even then.'

'It feels like a struggle to me.'

'Life is worth living – even when it's hard.'

'This hard?'

'It's worth living, because it's life.'

There is a beat of silence.

'Can I ask you another question?'

'If you must.'

'I've realised I don't know what it's been like for you.'

'What?'

'The tests. The treatment. Ejaculating in a cupboard.'

'I don't think about it.'

'I think I thought that.'

'That's because you're good at thinking. You can think for two.'

Another beat of silence.

'You still haven't told me how you feel.'

'Mostly I feel sad about the situation.'

'And what else?'

'Helpless. Sometimes I feel helpless.'

'Why?'

'Because I can't give you what you deserve.'

'Do I deserve it?'

'Everyone deserves to be happy.'

'And what about you?'

'I'm happy when you're happy.'

Another beat.

'Do you think we'll ever make love for fun again?'

'I hope so.'

'I hope so too.'

Silence.

Shift Happens

People often say they're fed up with their life and then do nothing about it – it's a very human trait. How many times have you heard friends say they want out of a relationship or a job, but then they don't do anything to change the situation? The truth is, we're quick to say we've had enough of something before we really have. But when we have had enough, when the camel's back is truly broken, most of us do something about it. Shift happens.

I have now been trying to have a baby for nearly six years. I have been through seven cycles of IVF. Five full and two frozen. I have had three biochemical pregnancies, one ectopic, and a miscarriage. The other two cycles were negative (well, presumed negative, as I started to bleed and didn't bother to take a test). This, along with turning forty, is what it takes for me to stop saying that something has to change in my life and actually do something about it.

For a while now I have been rotating round a circle of wondering whether the pressure of my job is affecting my fertility and whether I should give it up; then wondering what I'd do if I forfeited my career and didn't get pregnant. But shortly after my fortieth birthday and our seventh round of unsuccessful IVF, I decide to ask the chairman of my theatre if I can take a three-month sabbatical.

A couple of friends have suggested the idea to me over the years but I have constantly dismissed it out of guilt and, if I'm honest, fear of finding out that nobody needs me, not even work. However, I also know that the only person who will deny me a break is myself, and a sabbatical seems the perfect opportunity to take one without having to consider the drastic step of leaving altogether to pursue something that I might ultimately have no control over. So I swallow all my guilt, fear and pride, and ask for one.

And there's more. We decide to rent out our house in Oxford and move back to London. It is almost three years to the day since we moved in, and three years plus a week since I realised the move was probably a mistake. Whilst it did have the desired effect of stopping me from spending so much time at work, I simply swapped the office for a four-hour commute instead. I soon found myself regularly catching the train at 6.30 in the morning, getting home at midnight after an evening event, only to be back on the train first thing the following day. It felt like I was travelling a hundred miles a day just to go to sleep; it was exhausting and miserable.

With hindsight I do wonder why a moderately intelligent couple (us) would go away for the weekend; put an offer in on a house that they've seen only once in a city where they don't know anyone; and then borrow hundreds of thousands of pounds to buy it. But I guess impulse took over, along with a need to have control over something in our lives to counter the other thing over which we seem to have no control at all.

London is a city of villages, and one of the most exciting things about coming back is deciding where to move to. I've lived north, south, east and west, and have favourite places in every area. However, I quickly decide that I am determined to be as central as possible. So we swap our three-bedroom house in Oxford for a tiny top-floor one-bedroom flat in Covent Garden. It's heaven in a shoebox.

Friends just laugh and say, 'Jessica! Only you!'

It's true, there aren't many people who would even contemplate moving to the centre of touristville, and admittedly it hasn't got the boho-chic of north and west, nor the contemporary cool of south and east. But let me extol its virtues, just for a moment. It takes a maximum of thirty minutes to get to nearly anywhere in the city. Most nights out are only a ten-minute stroll home. And anything you could possibly need is within five minutes of your doorstep. It also has a unique sense of community, in that it's a place where people live, work and visit. At 8 a.m. on a Monday it is full of people on their way to the office; at 8 p.m. on a Friday it's full of people out on the razzle; and then first thing on a weekend morning the streets are deserted and you have the place to yourself. I love the juxtaposition of the buzz and the quiet. I love the anonymity. I even love hearing people walking drunkenly home through the streets in the middle of the night. It makes me feel that all is right with the world.

So, we are back in London and I have put in motion plans to take a sabbatical. Now all we need to do is decide what to do next in our quest for a baby. Like locusts, we've already eaten our way through three of the top clinics in the country and we're still hungry. The question is, can anybody satisfy us? Every doctor we see says that there is nothing at all to indicate that we can't and won't get pregnant. Our consultant in Oxford has often said that, all things being equal, his recommendation would be to keep trying and eventually, by the law of probability, we will succeed. But I'm not a machine, and years of unsuccessful IVF take their physical, emotional and financial toll. I'm not ready to give up, but if we are going to go through it yet again I need to try something different, somewhere different.

It's time to try Taranissi.

Dr Mohammed Taranissi is one of the most successful, but also one of the most controversial, fertility doctors in the UK. In 2007, the BBC produced a *Panorama* programme about him in which he was accused of administering costly and unproven treatments. These include the consumption of large quantities of milk; daily blood analysis; and the practice of immune therapy using unlicensed products – he is one of the few doctors in the UK who administers the treatments pioneered by the Californian doctor that our consultant in Oxford had told us about. Much of this is frowned on by the medical establishment, and Professor Lord Winston – the nice man off the telly who is one of the country's most famous fertility specialists – went so far as to say: 'He makes you weep for the medical profession.'

The *Panorama* programme caused a massive furore and even resulted in a police raid on

Taranissi's premises. All the charges against him were eventually dropped, but he is still regarded with a lot of suspicion, despite his phenomenal success rates, which, according to the HFEA (the UK's independent regulator of fertility treatment), are practically double the national average. When I quizzed our consultant in Oxford about the practice of immune therapy, he told us that he was, in fact, one of the people who was sent in by the authorities to investigate Taranissi after the police raid. Whilst he said that he didn't believe that his approach could be advocated on any medical grounds, he also said he had come to accept that Taranissi had utter conviction in what he did and that the care at the clinic was unparalleled.

At our follow-up appointment after our last unsuccessful round of IVF, I decided to ask our consultant again whether he thought I should go to see Taranissi for another opinion.

'Jessica, if you're asking me whether I think you have a better chance of getting pregnant there than anywhere else then the answer is no,' he said. 'But if you're asking me whether I think you should try everything so that you don't have any regrets later then the answer would have to be yes.'

It was good advice. The important thing is that when you get to the end of the line – and only you know when you're there – you can look in your heart and know you've given it everything. Je ne regrette rien.

So one day, on my way back to the office after a meeting, I decide to take a detour and pay a visit to 13 Upper Wimpole Street, home of Mr Taranissi's clinic – the ARGC – to make an appointment. I don't tell Peter I'm going. I know he won't approve, as he leans to the side of the medical establishment and is convinced this man is a quack who is just after our money. As I walk along the street to the clinic, it feels like I'm on my way to see a lover with whom I am having a clandestine affair. I am paranoid that someone will see me and wonder what the hell I'm doing in Marylebone on a Thursday lunchtime.

I reach the building, a tall Georgian town house with a rather-scruffy looking blue door. I ring on the bell and the door buzzes open. Although I'm now used to the oddness of fertility clinics, I'm not in the least prepared for the surprise of what's behind it. From the outside it looks quiet and unassuming, but inside it is full of people: in the hall, in the waiting room, up the stairs and queuing out of the reception room at the back. It has not been nicknamed the 'Argy Bargy' for nothing. It's extraordinary. Scores of women (and a few men) of all ages and races, all there for the same thing. A baby.

I fill out a registration form and within a few weeks we are sent a date for an appointment. I decide to wait until the weekend before coming clean with Peter.

'Shall we go out for breakfast?' I say as soon as we wake up on Saturday morning.

'Sounds nice. I assume you have somewhere in mind.'

'What about the café at the end of the road?' I say. 'The one that does an Italian version of a full English – it's got the best sausages I've ever tasted.'

He smiles: 'You love being back in London, don't you?'

'What's not to love?' I reply.

Later, after I've polished off my plateful, I decide to broach the 'T' subject.

'Have you got your diary with you?' I say, trying to sound nonchalant.

'Why?' Peter says immediately. 'What have you gone and organised for us?'

'I was just wondering what you're doing on Thursday afternoon in two weeks' time.'

'I'm busy,' he says suspiciously without even opening his diary.

'Not to worry then,' I say.

I turn back to the Saturday newspaper, knowing full well he won't be able to leave it at that.

'Why?' he says.

'Why what?' I say, looking up.

'Why do you want to know what I'm doing that afternoon?'

'I just wondered whether you'd be free to do something with me.'

'What?'

'Just something. But don't worry if you're not free.'

'Well I might be free,' he says, reaching for his diary. 'If you tell me what it is.'

'It's just that I've made an appointment to see someone.'

'Not that dodgy doctor you've been going on about,' he says instantly, closing it again.

'That dodgy doctor has the best results in the country,' I say. 'He could be our last hope.'

After another two cups of tea and a long discussion he reluctantly agrees to come. I know he doesn't approve, but I also know that this comes from wanting to protect me. When I am sent off for the immune tests – which involve taking twelve vials of blood and over a grand from my credit card – he is convinced that they are going to diagnose that I've got all the problems possible. Not because he believes I've got any immune issues but because he thinks that's how they make their money.

When the results come back and say that my immune system looks more or less fine he has to start eating those thoughts. I, however, feel a bit mixed about these results. On the one hand, I'm pleased that things appear to be normal; on the other hand, I was secretly hoping it might finally provide an answer to our problems.

With the test results back, the clinic says that we can start treatment as soon as we like. But this time I'm doing things differently. I plan to start midway through my three-month sabbatical, giving myself a month to relax and get super healthy (five-a-day, eight-a-night, supplements, acupuncture, moderate-exercise, no-alcohol type of healthy). This will then leave a month for the treatment itself, and a month to adjust to the result. Positive or negative.

The Indigestion Diaries (A postscript)

Yes, you read that right. The Indigestion Diaries. It's not a typo. It's a one-off, special entry because I'm figuring you might want to know what happened on that front. Well, my indigestion symptoms continued on and off for over three years. I never found out what was wrong but I learned to manage it – mainly by making sure I didn't eat much at night, which did have the rather nice side-effect of making me lose a bit of weight for a while without even trying. It wasn't worth it though, not for the occasional agony. Then, almost as suddenly as it appeared, my indigestion disappeared, practically on the day that I organised my sabbatical and we moved back to London. It's now been several months and I haven't had a sign of it. I can happily eat a three-course dinner of potted prawns (in clarified butter) followed by steak and chips (with lashings of béarnaise sauce), followed by chocolate pudding (with cream or ice cream depending on the mood). Not even a twinge. It does make me wonder whether my body has been living some sort of double life.

PRICE PRITCHETT

I got home from work today to find a book on my pillow. Powder-blue with a black spine. The title: *Hard Optimism* by Price Pritchett.

'What's this?' I ask.

'A present,' Peter replies.

It's easy to argue against the merits of optimism if you're going through IVF. Whatever way you look at it the statistics aren't good. If you're under thirty-five you've got a 33 per cent chance of success, and this drops to 13 per cent once you're past forty. You're probably more likely to win on the Grand National. This is good news for pessimists like me who are never happier than when imagining the worst. As far as I'm concerned, pessimism is the best protection from high-risk situations (i.e. IVF) and inevitable disappointment (i.e. IVF and me) – it's basically the art of thinking it won't work, so that when it doesn't you're not as upset as you might have been had you thought it would.

Price Pritchett, on the other hand, doesn't set any store by the pessimist's logic. For him, fortune favours those who are optimistic, and the good news for me is that this is a skill that can be learned if it doesn't come naturally (which it doesn't). His unique take on optimism is that it's more than positive thinking; it's the art of non-negative thinking, especially when you're experiencing difficulties, failures, uncertainty and loss. So that's me and the other 87 per cent of post-forty IVFers then.

In Price's own words: 'Optimism or pessimism – ultimately it's your choice. You get to decide how you want to frame events. You choose how you'll interpret circumstances. Each of us is the engineer of our emotional life, the architect of our own happiness. Change the way you look at life, and you literally shape a different life for yourself.'

Take IVF as an example. Granted, it's not the way that anyone would ideally choose to have a baby, but there have been studies which show that families with children conceived by IVF are happier than those with children conceived naturally. The thinking behind this is that if you've had to go to extreme lengths to get something that you want then you appreciate it so much more once you've got it. So rather than being pessimistic about the process, Price would say I should turn my infertility into a positive. I have to admit it's quite a nice thought that the harder we try to have a baby, the happier we might eventually be.

Price Pritchett soon becomes the other man in our relationship. Every morning in bed over a pot of a tea, Peter reads me a chapter of the book. Thereafter, whenever I show signs of giving in or giving up he says, 'What would Price say?'

Price would say: 'Things turn out best for people who make the best of the way things turn out.'

Practise it.

The Infertility Diaries Part XVIII

Every time I start another round of IVF I count forward nine months and work out when I'm going to give birth. An autumn birth is good as it means our child will be the oldest in the academic year (and by default the cleverest). December or August is bad as I don't want to inflict the 'joint Christmas and birthday present' or 'everyone's on holiday and can't come to your party' scenarios on them. Then I start planning Baby Number 2. I'm not going to wait long, even if it means it will be a lot of work with two toddlers under three. This is if I don't have twins, which, of course, is a distinct possibility with IVF. Yes, I'm a pessimist, and I go into every round of IVF thinking it probably won't work. But I'm also a fertility fantasist, planning a future that might never happen. Welcome to my schizophrenic world.

INADEQUATE

The alarm rings, which means it's 5 a.m. I lean over in the darkness, feeling for the button to switch it off, then turn over, snuggle into Peter's back and close my eyes.

'Come on,' Peter says. 'You don't want to be late.'

'I'm starting to think this is a really bad idea,' I say, sleepily.

'What? Your sabbatical?'

'No, thinking it was a good idea to do what I'm about to do on the first day of it. I should have given myself a bit more time to wind down.'

'This might be the only way to make you wind down,' he says.

The thing that I am about to do is an eight-day residential course known as the Hoffman Process. I first heard about it nine months ago at the anger management weekend I went on after my miscarriage.

On the last day Mike, the course tutor, looked me in the eyes and said: 'Jessica, you need to do some work on your inner child. Otherwise she's going to bring you to your knees.'

'Really?' I said. 'How do I go about doing that?'

I wasn't sure what my inner child was or, indeed, whether I had any interest in getting to know her, but I did want to know more. He said it with such conviction, it felt as if he knew something I didn't.

It was Mike and that moment that led me to the Hoffman Process. As soon as I got home I googled it. Created by an eccentric American psychotherapist called Bob Hoffman in the 1960s, the process has slowly spread across the world and has been running in the UK for the last fifteen years. Bob, following in Freud and Jung's footsteps, believed that our childhood, and particularly our relationship with our parents, is hugely significant in the way our adult life plays out. His unique theory is that in early childhood we are our true selves, but we soon start to emulate the negative behaviours of our parents in order to earn their love. He describes this as the 'negative love syndrome'. By identifying these negative patterns and releasing the anger and shame around them, we are able to find our true selves again.

The website said that they held regular open meetings in London to provide potential participants with further information. So one late October evening I made my way to the college in the centre of Regent's Park to find out more. What had I got to lose? I arrived just before the proceedings were about to start and carefully avoided the woman behind a desk at the front of the room who was taking people's names. I slipped into a seat at the back of the Victorian classroom and slouched down into the collar of my winter coat.

The room was fairly full and quite a few people seemed to know each other, hugging as if they were old friends and quickly locking into animated conversation. After about ten minutes a man stood up at the front of the classroom. He was in his fifties and wearing a leather necklace with a silver pendant. Hmmm I thought: a bit new age, a bit happy clappy. This isn't going to be for me. I looked over at the door but quickly assessed that I was going to have to stick it out unless I was prepared for everyone to see me get up and leave – which I wasn't.

The man in the silver pendant started to explain the format of the evening. He said that it was both a welcome home session for those people who had just completed the process, and an information session for people who were interested in finding out more. This explained why so many people seemed to know each other. He then asked if anyone who had just completed the course would be prepared to stand up and say why they had done it and what their experience had been.

What happened next was extraordinary.

One by one people spontaneously came to the front of the room and spoke, almost evangelically, about what they had been through. A woman in her thirties who said she'd never been able to sustain a relationship and she finally understood why. A man who said he'd decided to do it when he woke up on his kitchen floor after yet another night's drinking and now had the strength to turn his life around. A woman who said she had done a lot of therapy and had initially been very cynical but had to admit it was the most amazing experience she had ever had in her life. And even a female Buddhist monk who said that it was the closest she'd got to enlightenment in years. I couldn't quite believe what I was hearing. This was either the best-executed marketing campaign I had ever seen or I was witnessing something that was real. If it was real, I wanted some of what they had just had.

I didn't sign up that evening. With our debt already out of control as a result of so many rounds of IVF (and that trip to the Point), I wasn't sure that I could justify the cost. It sounded good but would it help me get pregnant? Did I honestly think that my childhood could have anything to do with my infertility thirty years later? I wasn't sure, but the evening, and particularly the testimonies from those people who had just completed the process, kept playing over in my mind. So, a few weeks before I was due to finish work, I phoned and booked myself on to the course starting on 1 April. Day One of my sabbatical.

As per usual, we're late setting off. Peter's pushing ninety on the speedometer and I've got my feet up on the dashboard and am painting my toenails. I've been told to arrive by 9.30 a.m. At twenty-five minutes past, I ring to say I'm going to be a bit late. The Irishwoman who answers the phone says, rather tersely, that they'll be starting the first session at 10 a.m. on the dot. At 9.59 we swing into the driveway of the country house where the course is taking place. Peter takes my case out of the boot, hurriedly kisses me goodbye, and then leaves me on the doorstep for a week in the company of strangers.

There are sixteen of us on the course. We file into a large room at the back of the house overlooking the garden. Sixteen chairs are laid out in a semicircle, each bearing a folder with a name on it. I find my folder and sit down with relief. When the group has settled, the first thing we are asked to do is go round the circle and tell everyone what we are feeling at that moment.

When it's my turn I say: 'I'm just feeling pleased that I managed to get here on time.'

Everyone laughs.

Later that afternoon I have a one-to-one session with the man who is going to be my personal tutor for the week. He looks like Colin Firth. It's a bit distracting.

'So, Jessica,' he says. 'I couldn't help but notice that you didn't answer honestly this morning when we asked you all to say how you were feeling.'

'Didn't I?' I say. 'I mean, it was an honest answer but perhaps not the only answer.'

'I think you're someone who feels like you've got to protect yourself and your real feelings from other people. Look at your body language now, for example; it says a lot.'

I realise that my legs are not only crossed away from him but round the side of my chair, and that my left hand is holding my right shoulder, bringing my arm into a v-shape across my chest. A bit of a giveaway really.

We carry on talking. He has obviously read the pre-course questionnaire I completed, thoroughly, and acknowledges how hard the last six years must have been. I bat it away lightly, nowhere near ready to go there.

Towards the end of our session, he says: 'Before we finish, Jessica, I need to ask you to chose another name which you're going to be known by this week.'

I look at him, bemused. 'Another name?'

'Having read your questionnaire, I do have a couple of suggestions.'

'You do?'

'Yes,' he says. 'How about "Inadequate"?'

'Inadequate?' I say incredulously.

'It seems to fit.'

'Does it?'

'I think so.'

'Are you seriously suggesting that I go round with the word "Inadequate" pinned to my chest for the week?' I ask. 'I just couldn't. I just really couldn't.'

I can sense the panic in my voice.

'Well I do have some others,' he says. 'But, having met you, I'm not sure they're right.'

He tells me what they are and slowly, reluctantly, I agree that of all the choices he has presented, 'Inadequate' most closely resonates with my relationship with the world and how I feel about being unable to have a baby. He asks me to give him the badge I am wearing which says 'Jessica', pulls out the piece of white card with my name on it, turns it over, and writes 'Inadequate' on the other side. Then he slips it back into its plastic case, the right way up, so my new name is hidden.

Relieved, I put it back on.

Amongst other things, we had been told to bring to the course a picture of ourselves as a child, aged five or six. For the last session of the afternoon we are all asked to produce it. I have bought a school photograph of me with shoulder-length baby-blonde hair, wearing a bright yellow polo-neck jumper, a navy blue corduroy dress and a hairband made out of American Indian beads. I can't help thinking that if I had fallen pregnant when Peter and I first started trying to conceive, our child might be around this age now.

We all sit down holding our photographs and are asked to put them on the floor in front of us. The room settles into silence.

'Welcome back everyone,' the Course Director says. 'I hope you've had a good afternoon settling in.'

There is a murmur of assent.

'Earlier today in the session with your tutor each of you was given a new name,' she continues. 'We'd now like you to take off your badge, turn the card over to reveal it and then put it back on. After that, we will go round the circle and we want you to introduce yourself using your new name by saying, "I am _____".'

I can hear my heart thumping through my chest. I hardly know these people and haven't even had the opportunity to tell most of them my real name yet. The embarrassment is excruciating. I glance round and see that everyone is doing what they've been told, so I start to fumble with my own badge, wondering why the hell I'm putting myself through this. But there's no going back now. One by one, just as we've been told, we all formally introduce ourselves for the first time that day.

'I am I Don't Matter.'

'I am Unworthy.'

'I am Anxious.'

'I am On the Other Hand.'

'I am Fraud.'

'I am In My Bubble.'

'I am Let Down.'

'I am Alone and Lost.'

'I am Abandoned.'

'I am Not Good Enough.'

'I am Dismissed.'

'I am Fixer.'

'I am Lonely.'

'I am Controlled.'

'I am Unimportant.'

And:

'*I* am Inadequate.'

I look around the circle at my fellow participants, realising for the first time that every one of us has come to the course carrying a profound sense of pain. I don't know anything about these people or their lives, but I am not alone.

The Course Director then asks us to kneel down on the floor and crouch over our photographs.

'Get down close,' she urges. 'Look into your eyes in the photograph and think about your name. Ask yourself why this child, so innocent and so beautiful, got to feel like that.'

Out of the corner of my eye I can see people crouching down. I start to hear sobbing on my left and my right. But I can't move, frozen with fear of what might happen if I get down close and look into the eyes of my five-year-old self. So I sit back, holding on to tears, knowing that whatever happens over the next seven days it's going to be important in my journey to have a child.

The Infertility Diaries Part XIX

On the final day of the Hoffman Process, our tutor asked us to think back to the day we all met and try to remember the first impressions we had of each other and whether they had changed. The woman who sat next to me throughout the process turned to me and said: 'The first time I saw you, you seemed like a mother to me. You still do.' Everyone immediately agreed. And, for the first time in a long time, I actually believed it could be true.

Thoughts on Therapy

Now for a fertility fact. Fertility clinics – however high their success rates – are crap at the psychological stuff. Well that's my experience anyway. When you receive your glossy brochure/photocopied sheets of A4 about the clinic, you'll generally find a (small) section on 'counselling'. It's usually just a few sentences about the emotional impact of fertility treatment, and if you're lucky you might be offered a counselling session. But in all my years of going through this, I haven't yet found a clinic or consultant that has ever proactively encouraged us to take up that session or asked what we're doing to sort out our minds.

At our first clinic we did ask if we could have one. The staff looked as if they'd never been asked before, but with a bit of faffing an appointment was eventually arranged. As nice as the lady who saw us was, let's just say she wasn't prepared for me and my neuroses. When I told her about my paranoia that the clinic was going to mix up my eggs with someone else's sperm, I could see her thinking: this woman has some serious issues. Absolutely right, and one session wasn't even going to scratch the surface.

Whether or not the Hoffman Process could have any direct impact on my next round of treatment, I'm sure it's been important. During the first few days we were not allowed to talk to each other about the things one would usually talk about with strangers. So, for once, I didn't tell anyone what my job was or whether or not I had children, and nobody asked. One of the peculiar things about this was that it made me realise how much I use my work to validate myself, particularly in the context of not being a mother. It helped me to discover who I was beyond work and, crucially, beyond my infertility. Gradually, I came to realise that all the negative feelings I have about my life, particularly in the context of my inability to have a child, do not accurately represent me, or, in fact, what other people think of me. It took away a lot of shame.

I now firmly believe that everybody needs therapy every now and again (the time to worry is when you find yourself in it for the rest of your life). We all have our shit. And if your shit's infertility, you're going to need it more than most.

The Infertility Diaries Part XX

My friend Ella gave me a great piece of advice today. She says it's all about the number forty-three. If you haven't had children by then you can basically get on with the rest of your life and stop thinking about it. It's quite a liberating and exciting thought. I've got three years left and, if it doesn't work out, after that I can go off and become an astronaut. Or something.

M R   T

I am now halfway through my sabbatical. It's amazing what can happen in six weeks. We've had a royal wedding; Osama bin Laden's been killed; and Bruce Forsyth has finally been knighted. As for me, I'm ready to start my first round of IVF with Mr Taranissi. It's been a long time coming, and I'm feeling a mixture of excitement and trepidation.

In IVF there are essentially two treatment types: the long protocol and the short protocol. The long protocol involves down-regulating your body before stimulation starts, and the short protocol works with your natural cycle. Up until now I have always had the long one, but the short protocol is often considered to be better for older women (which, at forty, I am now classed as being) and this is what Mr Taranissi has prescribed in my case. It also has the added benefit of taking slightly less time – around a month from beginning to end – and I have worked out a schedule for my sabbatical which means I will be able to complete my treatment a few weeks before I'm due back at work.

I have been told by the clinic that I will need to come in for a blood test on either the first or second day of my period. It started yesterday afternoon and, as it's a sunny Sunday morning, I decide to walk to the clinic. Peter is away working so I'm on my own.

After a thirty-minute stroll I arrive at Upper Wimpole Street. As I go into the reception room I catch a glimpse of Mr Taranissi (fondly known by staff and patients as 'Mr T') in the hallway in blue scrubs. This man may be making a lot of money, but you have to admire anyone who is prepared to work seven days a week to make so many women's dreams come true.

I wait in line for the form on which all blood tests at the clinic are prescribed. The blood is taken at another building around the corner, and throughout the day there is a constant stream of women going from one building to the other with their distinctive yellow slips fluttering in the breeze. When I reach the blood-test building I find the door open, and am confronted by what can only be described as a sea of women. I can't quite believe that they are all Taranissi's patients, but they seem to be holding yellow forms like mine so they must be. It's like some sort of surreal baby-making factory. I feel a woman who has come in behind me squeeze past and pick up a laminated ticket from the counter. Then another woman does the same. There is clearly a protocol, which I'm about to learn. I reach over and take a ticket myself. Number 73!

A woman comes out from the back and calls: 'Numbers 20, 21, 22, 23, 24 and 25, please come through.'

I'm going to be in for a wait.

I hadn't quite realised the importance of this blood test until I'd rung the clinic to let them know I was planning to start treatment on my next cycle. It had been several months since I had my initial consultation and tests, and it was only when I rang that they said that they would need to check my FSH (or to give it its proper name: follicle stimulating hormone) to confirm that I could start. When I asked why, they said that Mr Taranissi will generally only let you start treatment if your FSH is under 10, because it is a strong indicator of the quality of your eggs and the likelihood of success. I hadn't even contemplated the possibility that there might be a situation where I wouldn't be able to start when I wanted to. This had never happened at my previous clinics. But like many aspects of the fertility process, knowledge reveals itself to you slowly.

After a three-hour wait for the results, the phone rings. It appears my FSH is fine, but another hormone, oestradiol, is on the high side. I am told to come back the following day for a further blood test and another nail-biting wait. The next day my oestradiol has increased. This essentially means that one follicle is starting to out-strip all the others, as it would on a natural cycle with a view to producing one egg. I am told that Mr Taranissi says I need to come back next month and go through the process again.

This is not a good moment. In fact, it's a really bad one. It is almost a year since my last round of IVF, and I have planned for my sabbatical and this cycle with meticulous precision. I am due back at work in six weeks and, although I have always known that the treatment might not be successful, I had never contemplated that I might not be able to start at all. But I can also see the sense of it. Here is a clinic that isn't going to put me through treatment if they don't think I stand the best chance of success. That's got to be a good thing. It also defies any cynicism that Mr Taranissi is just after our money. So I do my best to make a positive out of a negative, and we go on lastminute.com and book a cheap holiday to Madrid for a week of tapas, cerveza and the Prado.

Price would be proud.

One month later: the moment my period starts we're back at the clinic. FSH fine. Oestradiol still behaving badly. A decision is made to give me a down-regulation injection for a few days to bring it under control. I'm anxious that again things are not going to plan, but I'm assured it's completely normal and that my oestradiol levels will soon be stable and I'll be ready to start. Just to prove that nothing is ever simple where my body is concerned, a few days later it has quintupled. Yes, that's right. Gone up five flipping times. So now they put me into full down-regulation mode, trying to bring on a period as quickly as possible so we can start all over again. It feels as if my body's screaming: 'WHAT THE HELL ARE YOU DOING TO ME?' And, just to prove what it's talking about, two weeks later when my oestradiol has finally been beaten into submission and my system shut down, I have a scan and there's an enormous cyst in one of my ovaries.

Ovarian cyst – two words that would have any woman running screaming to the Internet. Apparently, though, the majority of them are benign and self-combust naturally. The doctor who scans me doesn't seem at all perturbed, but I do feel sorry for my body and what I am putting it through. Again.

Later the same evening, five weeks behind my carefully planned schedule, I finally get the call I've been waiting for. Mr Taranissi has confirmed that he's happy for me to start treatment. I am told to come in for a hysteroscopy in two days' time, after which they will start stimulation. I haven't had one of these before as it's not something that is routinely done during fertility treatment, but of course, with this as with everything else, Mr T is different. The procedure is performed under general anaesthetic and involves an investigation of my uterus to make sure everything is looking normal and to work out the best place to put our embryos back. In my case it also involves the aspiration of a certain cyst.

The day of the procedure marks a new chapter in my fertility journey. It's the day I get to go to the basement. For some time now, I've been aware of the stairs that lead to the lower ground floor of the clinic that only a select few of the women in the waiting room get to descend. It's the inner sanctum of the fertility process, the place where eggs are collected and embryos are transferred. And also where hysteroscopies happen. My moment has arrived.

Although I've seen a few clinics by now, I have to say that I've never experienced anything quite like it. Generally you get your own cubicle. Sometimes you get your own room. But here you lie side by side with all the other patients, waiting to go into theatre and then recovering alongside them afterwards. It's strange to think back now on my first ever experience of a fertility clinic: my paranoia about my eggs being mixed with someone else's sperm, and my horror at being treated in a hospital corridor. Now, years later, I succumb silently to this factory line in what feels like some sort of Orwellian nightmare (although this is a nightmare in which all I want is for my dream to come true).

Following an all-clear from my hysteroscopy I move on to the stimulation phase. This is also nothing like I've experienced anywhere before. Each morning I have to go into the clinic for a blood test and every other day I have a scan. I then wait for a call to tell me my daily drug dose. Every day it's different, and the instructions are incredibly specific, ranging from take it 'NOW' to take it tomorrow morning at exactly 5 a.m. Added to this there's the two litres of water and litre of milk I have to drink each day. I seem to be spending the whole time rushing to public toilets either to have a pee or to shoot up.

During the latter stages of stimulation the blood tests and scans increase to two per day, all in a bid to pinpoint the perfect moment to trigger ovulation.

It's an exhausting but exhilarating process, which takes over my life. I'm just thankful that I have swallowed my secrecy about what I'm doing on my sabbatical and arranged to take another month off work.

The majority of the medical profession consider Taranissi's obsession with the minutiae unnecessary. Much of his practice is still clinically unproven. His daily regime of blood tests and drug concoctions is also what makes treatment here double the price of anywhere else. But, having been through this process multiple times now, the one thing that it does make you feel is that you are receiving treatment that is tailor-made for you. Maybe it's not the blood tests and drugs but the level of care that yields his results. Either way, it's got to be worth it.

Midway through the second week of stimulation I get the call I've been longing for. I am called in for a scan with Mr T himself. It's the first time I've met him in person and it's a bit like meeting God. Not because I'm yet convinced that he will succeed where others have failed, but because of the omnipotent authority with which he runs the clinic. No decision is made on any patient's treatment without his say-so, and he undertakes a lot of the egg collections and transfers himself. It's a level of commitment and care from a senior consultant that, in my experience, is unprecedented in the fertility industry.

'It's such a pleasure to meet you,' I gush.

It's just as well Peter's not here because I know he wouldn't approve of such sycophancy.

'Thank you. Thank you,' he says. 'So what do you do?'

'I work in a theatre,' and then add quickly for clarification: 'Not an operating theatre. A theatre where people perform.'

I've realised over the last few years that this definition is necessary when talking to medical professionals.

He smiles. 'And what clinic were you at before you came here?'

'Oh, a few. You're my last hope.'

'Ah, you should have come here first.'

'Probably,' I say. 'Everyone says that if anyone can get me pregnant, you can.'

He smiles again.

I can feel a miniature Peter on my shoulder saying that flattery won't necessarily get me a baby. Maybe not, but I can only try.

I lie silently on the trolley as he scans me. Usually I would be leaning over, peering at the screen to try to count the follicles myself, but today I am so in awe that I don't dare.

'Things are looking good,' Mr Taranissi says. 'I'll

need to review your blood results from this afternoon but we will probably trigger you tonight or tomorrow. Then, in nine months, you'll have a baby.'

I wonder how he can sound so confident, but I kind of like that he does.

The Infertility Diaries Part XXI

I have recently developed a condition that can only be described as Infertility Envy. I look at all the other women in the clinic and find a million reasons to be jealous of them. I envy the women with thin patient files who have only just started treatment and who I surmise will be successful on their first or second attempt. I envy the women with thicker files than mine, believing that their experience and determination will soon deliver results. When I'm waiting in the queue to have my blood taken, I strain to hear other women giving their date of birth, envious of all those who were born after 1970 and are younger than me. I'm envious of the women the receptionists seem to know and sometimes allow to jump the scan queue; and of the women who have forged friendships with other women and chat together in hushed tones about their treatment. And if all this weren't enough, I'm also envious about all the usual stuff – the women who are thinner, prettier and richer than me –

allowing myself to believe that these are all qualities that
make them more deserving of getting a baby than I am.
But of course in reality we are all the same. All of us have
been denied something that we desperately want. We are
equal in our infertility (even if in my envious eyes some
are more equal than others).

DORITOS (FAMILY SIZE)

On the day of egg collection we arrive at the clinic,
as instructed, at 6.30 a.m. It's a beautiful morning
which, after the week of rain that has preceded it,
feels like some sort of pathetic fallacy. A day of hope
and new beginning.

At seven o'clock, I am taken down to the
basement, and Peter is taken up to the producing
room. I have long since given up insisting on being
together for this bit of the process. Clinics just don't
get it and, in all honesty, I've realised it's probably
easier for Peter if I'm not around. Plus, at Mr
Taranissi's clinic there's such a long queue of men
waiting to produce each morning that speed is of the
essence. Later, Peter proudly tells me that he was in
and out of the room in a total of twelve minutes: a
new record.

There are six women having egg collection this

morning. I am Number 4. I get chatting to Numbers 3 and 5 on either side of me. Number 3 is a party planner from West London; Number 5 is a paediatrician from Reading.

'Is that hard?' I ask Number 5.

'Sometimes,' she says.

Only another woman living with infertility could ask this question of a stranger and understand how hard it must be.

One by one we are walked into theatre, then afterwards wheeled out on a trolley and lined up side by side in recovery. I have made a pact with myself that this time around I'm not going to ask *that* question as soon as I wake up. I will bide my time. The answer will come when it comes and will be what it will be.

Whilst I am sipping my post-op tea and eating digestive biscuits the answer is delivered to me on a sheet of paper. At the top it says: 'You have had eight eggs collected today.' It's fewer than I hoped for but more than our last cycle, which is now nearly a year ago. I guess I have to accept that, at forty, the heady days of double figures are over. Besides, they never got me pregnant, so it's not like the numbers actually meant anything anyway. As so many doctors have told me, all we need is one plus one – one good egg plus one good sperm.

As I'm sitting pondering this the paediatrician is

wheeled in next to me. As soon she wakes up I hear her ask the nurse: 'How many eggs?'

The next morning the news is that, of my eight eggs, six were mature and injectable; of these, five have fertilised. By Day 3 the development of two of them is slowing down, but three have reached eight cells and the decision is made to put them back. This is the first cycle I have had since turning forty and I am now eligible to have up to three embryos transferred. It seems a lot. Whilst I think most couples going through IVF would secretly be happy with twins (largely so they don't have to go through it all again), I'm not sure anyone can comprehend the thought of triplets. But I know the chances of this happening are minute, especially given our track record, so we go for the hat-trick.

It's now my third visit to the basement, and I'm starting to feel quite at home. Mr Taranissi does the transfer himself, chatting and joking at first, and then falling silent in complete concentration as he manoeuvres the catheter containing our embryos into my uterus. It's the longest transfer procedure I've had and it feels like he's taking the utmost care to put them back in exactly the right place. I like that.

Afterwards he tells us to wait upstairs whilst he reviews my medication for the next two weeks. The waiting room is unusually quiet. There are two women sitting on their own and an attractive young couple who are clearly here for their first consultation, busily filling out forms. The man's name is called by one of the receptionists and he is taken upstairs alone. He bounds in a while later with a smile on his face.

'Producing room,' I mouth at Peter.

'I was quicker,' he mouths back.

Then we are joined by a Moslem couple with three young children: a girl of about five, and a boy and girl of about three who are clearly twins. The wife is dressed in black burka from head to toe with only a tiny slit for her eyes. I smile at her, trying to tell whether she smiles back. I can't, but after a while she pulls out a big bag of Doritos, gives one to each of the children, and then offers the packet to me across the room. It's one of those special moments of connection across cultures, and as I take a crisp her husband suddenly says, pointing at the children:

'Taranissi. All of them. My wife and I tried for eighteen years. We went all over the world. But nothing. And then, Taranissi. All of them.'

'That's amazing,' I say.

Everyone in the room spontaneously agrees.

I can hardly imagine what it must have been like for this couple and for other couples that come from cultures where the woman's primary role in life is to bear children. It must have been terrible for them both that they couldn't. And eighteen years. It makes our six and a half feel like a breeze.

Then, as if the husband's confession has broken a spell over the room, everyone starts to share their own stories. Each one different and yet the same. It's such a rare moment in a fertility waiting room, usually loaded with uncomfortable silence. A reminder of how much we all want to know each other's experiences, and share our own, but how few opportunities there are to ask.

So begins another two-week wait. It's the first I've spent doing nothing. For all my other cycles I have carried on working and, to be honest, I don't know what's worse: waiting and doing something, or waiting and doing nothing. I think a lot about the other women who had their eggs collected on the same day, knowing that they will be going through exactly the same emotions as me. Monitoring every twinge, shifting between feeling positive and negative.

One of the strangely comforting things is that, unlike my previous clinics, Mr T still has me on a whole range of different drugs. Twice daily injections and a junior aspirin to thin the blood; a steroid tablet that has to be taken at exactly six-hour intervals, which involves waking up every morning at 4 a.m.; and a nightly injection of progesterone into my bottom. Nice. But it does feel like we're doing stuff to help the process and that's a comfort.

As usual, the first few days are easy as it's too early to get anxious about what is or isn't happening. But as the days count down I am increasingly torn between wanting the uncertainty to end and the hope to last forever. I have also made a second pact with myself (second to the not-asking-how-many-eggs pact), which is that I am not going to do my regular 'spot check'. The deal I've struck is that when I wipe I mustn't look, but I can take a quick glance in the toilet bowl before I flush the chain – just to make sure there isn't anything significant. This is going well, a small triumph in itself, and when I safely pass the day on which I usually start spotting I feel a sense of jubilation. Statistically speaking I have started spotting on all but one of my IVF attempts before official test day (and that time I was pregnant), so not spotting has got to be a good sign. A really good sign.

The Infertility Diaries Part XXII

I have become an infertility stalker. I spend hours on websites and blogs reading other people's conversations. I never sign up or log in, too embarrassed to officially declare myself.

I know I'm not alone. On one of my favourite stalking sites – Fertility Friends – it tells you how many guests and how many official users are online at any one time. Day or night there are always hundreds of people, many just voyeurs like me.

If I'm honest these sites scare me a bit. The women are all so knowledgeable and talk in acronyms that it took me a long time to understand. Now I'm scared by the fact that I'm starting to speak their language.

Me and DP TTC nearly 7yrs. Spent £££ on TX, OPK and Pee Sticks. Virtually given up on all BMS. DX U-IF. TX so far: IUI (disaster); ICSI (CP then BFN); FET (CP then BFN); ICSI (AF arrived. Didn't bother testing on OTD); ICSI (ditto); ICSI (BFN then DX ectopic); FET (BFP! then M/C 9wks): ICSI (CP then BFN); ICSI (D/R a muddle; stims OK; E/C Fri; E/T Mon; now on 2WW 9 DPT PUPO). AFM all I want is to get PG and have a DD or a DS. Is that TMTA?*

I think I might have actually just made up the acronym 'TMTA': too much to ask. Now I'm really scared. The stalker becomes the stalked.

[*Me and Dear Partner Trying To Conceive for nearly seven years. Spent thousands of pounds on Treatment, Ovulation Predicator Kits and Home Pregnancy Tests. Virtually given up on all Baby-Making Sex. Diagnosed with Unexplained Infertility. Treatment so far: Intrauterine Insemination (disaster); Intracytoplasmic Sperm Injection (Biochemical Pregnancy then Big Fat Negative); Frozen Egg Transfer (Biochemical Pregnancy then Big Fat Negative); Intracytoplasmic Sperm Injection (Aunt Flo arrived. Didn't bother testing on Official Test Date); Intracytoplasmic Sperm Injection (ditto); Intracytoplasmic Sperm Injection (Big Fat Negative then diagnosed with Ectopic Pregnancy); Frozen Egg Transfer (Big Fat Positive! Then Miscarriage at 9 weeks); Intracytoplasmic Sperm Injection (Biochemical Pregnancy then Big Fat Negative); Intracytoplasmic Sperm Injection (Down Regulation a muddle; Stimulation OK; Egg Collection Friday; Egg Transfer Monday; now on Two Week Wait, 6 Days Post Transfer, Pregnant Until Proven Otherwise). As For Me, all I want is to get Pregnant and have a Dear Daughter or a Dear Son. Is that Too Much To Ask?]

ZEBRAS AND LEOPARDS

I've decided to have my hair done this afternoon at a new salon just round the corner from us. It's in a beautifully restored Victorian town house with stripped wooden floors and Farrow & Ball paintwork. They even serve tea made with muslin teabags. The prospect of a hair makeover and a few hours reading glossy magazines seems like the perfect way to spend the afternoon before test day.

Everything is going well until the reveal. When the hairdresser swivels me round to show me the back of my head, I am horrified to see that it looks like a yellow and black zebra. Usually, like most women in the world, I would smile rigidly, hand over my credit card and race home in tears. But today I find myself exclaiming: 'But it's stripey!'

Within minutes all the stylists in the salon have come over and are running their fingers through my hair, saying it looks fabulous, whilst all the other customers are staring at me in pity, breathing a silent sigh of relief that it's not them. It doesn't look fabulous, it looks stripey, and no amount of primping can console me. But as the discussion escalates I become increasingly embarrassed that it ever began, and eventually do a bad job of telling the guy who cut it not to worry, pay and leave.

Peter meets me outside the salon and we have a tense walk home. Why is it that men will never learn that if a woman doesn't like her haircut no amount of saying it looks 'fine' will make it better? It actually makes it worse. I now feel terrible: for causing a scene; for probably ruining the day of the man who cut it; and for having to go out in stripes. Do I need a clearer sign that I am stressed about tomorrow –

either that or I've got pregnancy hormones racing around my body…

I have decided to do a test at home first thing in the morning, prior to going to the clinic for my official blood test. Mr Taranissi doesn't even give you the option of doing a home test (which, following my ectopic, I think is a very good thing). However, I've been giving it quite a bit of thought and have decided that by doing a test at home first, I'll get a heads up and this will make the wait for the blood test result marginally less agonising.

I sleep sporadically and in my waking moments mull over how to do the test. Shall I pee on it or collect the urine in a pot? The problem with the pee thing is that it often won't go where you want it to, and you find yourself chasing it around the toilet bowl as it goes everywhere but on the stick itself. As I've only bought one test I don't want to risk it. But the alternative is a pot, and what to use? I don't like the idea of peeing into a glass we'll be drinking from later. I mentally run through all the container-like objects in our flat that might fit the job, and finally land on the ball you put into the washing machine. I wonder whether the residue detergent might have an effect, but I guess it guarantees it's clean. That's settled, I think, and fall back to sleep for a few hours.

When I wake up again it's about ten to six. Peter

is still breathing heavily. I get up and head for the door. He looks up blearily.

'I'm going to do it,' I say.

Ball filled. Stick inserted for five seconds (plus another five for luck). I take the test back to bed and put it on the bedside table without looking at it. I check the clock: 05.59.

'Three minutes,' I say.

'OK,' Peter replies, stretching out of sleep.

At exactly 06.02 I pick up the test and hold it out in front of us. There is one clear pink line. We both look at it.

'Not pregnant,' I say. Almost in disbelief.

Peter is silent for a while.

'Maybe it's too early,' he says. 'We should wait for the results of the blood test from the clinic.'

'It won't make any difference,' I say. 'I'm *not* pregnant.'

I hold the test in my hand, staring at it. I was so sure that this time it was going to work. That this time our luck had finally changed.

Then I have an idea. I prise the stick open: it falls apart relatively easily in my hands. I take out the little strip where the test lines appear. I hold it up to the light and examine it for a trace of a second line, even a very faint one.

But there's nothing.

Then I start to wonder whether the test might be

faulty. My mind runs through all the possibilities. Perhaps I shouldn't have used the detergent ball. Perhaps they have forgotten to add the chemical that reacts with the pregnancy hormone. Perhaps there are other women out there like me with a false result due to a dodgy batch. But, at the same time, the slow slide into disappointment and despondency has begun.

I guess zebras sometimes change their stripes, but leopards never change their spots.

We are due at the clinic at nine but I persuade Peter that, for once, it won't matter if we're late. I want to avoid the other women who were with me at egg collection and who I know will all be testing on the same day. I don't want to have an awkward conversation in the corridor in which I blurt out that I've already done a test at home and the result was negative.

My plan works. When we arrive the clinic is empty, and I'm able to go in and out without seeing anyone.

Afterwards we walk to Regent's Park and sit on a bench in the sun, waiting for the call. After two and a half hours it comes. The moment I answer I can tell from the way the nurse says 'hello' what she's going to say. I ask her if there is any of the HCG pregnancy hormone in my blood at all, wondering – almost wishing – whether at the very least it might be another biochemical pregnancy. But she says there's nothing. Not a trace.

Even my most pessimistic self can't understand how after everything – the daily blood tests, scans and injections; the litre of milk and two of water; the extra supplements and acupuncture that I've been having on the side; Hoffman; and, of course, my sabbatical – that the result is negative. That it's all been for absolutely nothing.

We sit in silence. I can hear the trickle of a fountain over to the right of us; the sun is warming my face; but my internal world has stopped with the shock and sadness that this is happening to us yet again.

The next day I start the process of telling people, by text and email. Family, friends, colleagues. So many people now know what we've been going through and that it has been one of the main reasons for my sabbatical. It's hard and the last thing I want to do, but I know they'll be waiting for the result.

The phone rings. It's Beth. As soon as I pick up, she bursts into tears. Another friend sends me a text, urging me not to give up and saying she wants to organise a fundraiser to raise the money for us to try again. I am so touched by their concern and friendship. But how could I ever agree when people would probably just be throwing their money away.

I am due to start back at work tomorrow. I can't put

it off any longer, having already taken five weeks more than I was supposed to. The saddest thing is that all the happy memories of the last few months are difficult to hold on to now that the foremost reason for taking my sabbatical has failed. I lie awake all night thinking everything over. Just before I started treatment I had coffee with a friend of a friend who had been through multiple rounds of failed IVF at other clinics and had got pregnant with Mr Taranissi first time. She enthused about his clinic and said that she had met lots of people who had been there and that every one of them got pregnant. I remember saying how I hoped I wasn't going to be the first person to let her down. But of course I am. Just in case I'd forgotten, good luck and miracles are what happen to other people.

I try to imagine what the rest of my life might be like: never experiencing what it feels like to be fat with pregnancy; never getting to feel that first kick of life inside me; never being able to say 'I think my waters have broken' (never even knowing what that really means); never being told to push by a kindly midwife; never being able to shout legitimately for gas and air; never having a newborn baby placed on my chest and saying hello for the first time.

After a while I become aware that Peter is lying awake next to me.

'What do you think we should do now?' I ask. 'Is it time to give up?'

'Is that what you want?'

'Of course not. I don't want to accept that the last six and a half years have all been for nothing. But then I think about what not giving up means. Another round of: How many follicles? How many eggs? How many fertilised? Then the dreaded two-week wait. The fear of spotting. Now the fear of not spotting. I'm just not sure that I can do it any more.'

'It's hard,' he says. 'And unfair.'

'So what do you think we should do?

'I think we only give up when there's no more hope. There's still hope.'

We fall asleep in each other's arms. When I wake up I feel light, but within moments consciousness takes over, and with it an overwhelming sense of sadness.

But there's no time to dwell on it. It's Monday morning and back to school.

The Infertility Diaries Part XXIII

Beyoncé is having a baby. She said she'd become a mother at thirty. She's now twenty-nine and a half so her timing's perfect. Unlike me, she was clearly the '-est' of a lot of things at school: the prettiest, the talented-est, definitely the luckiest. The Evening Standard *runs an article with the headline*

'30 THINGS TO DO BEFORE YOU'RE 30'. Item Number 2 reads:

> *HAVE A BABY (IF YOU'RE A WOMAN)*
> *We've all read those scary news stories – surely every 29-year-old is quaking with infertility fear? Now Beyoncé, our top role model, has got herself pre-30 pregnant. Time to follow suit.*

Good advice, I'd say.

SHOW ME THE EVIDENCE

In addition to IVF I have tried most alternative therapies associated with infertility. Acupuncture. Homeopathy. You name it; I've been there. I haven't just got the T-shirt, I've got one in every colour.

A few years after we started trying for a baby, someone recommended an acupuncturist to me who she was convinced had helped her to conceive. There's nothing as persuasive as a personal recommendation so Peter and I both went to see her.

I have never got over how odd it feels to lie on a couch and have needles stuck into you. It's not that they hurt – they are more like tiny pins than needles

– it's more that I can't quite understand what they can actually be doing, as they hardly puncture the skin. The session would always start with her feeling my pulse and saying wise and weird things like, 'Your yin is working hard today,' or, 'Your spleen is a bit sluggish.' I wanted to believe it meant something but I could never really persuade myself that it did.

After each session Peter and I would compare notes.

'How many needles did you have today?' I'd ask.

'Oh, I don't know, about fifteen,' he'd reply.

'Fifteen! That's not fair. I only had two. Where did she put them?'

'Well, I had three in each ear…'

'In your ears? I only ever get a couple in my hands and feet. Sometimes my stomach if I'm lucky.'

'Maybe my need is greater.'

'Maybe you're just getting special treatment,' I harrumphed.

Despite my ongoing competition with Peter about numbers of needles, I enjoyed my visits to Ann the acupuncturist. She had that motherly quality that a lot of alternative therapists have, and it made me relax as soon as I arrived. She was also a cranial therapist, and would sit at the top of the table and hold my head whilst the needles did their thing. I could never work out what this did either but it felt nice. I often wonder whether she had some psychic-like power and just by feeling my pulse or touching my head she could tell what was going on in my body and why I wasn't able to conceive. If she did, she never said.

So if acupuncture alone couldn't help me, maybe something else could. The next thing I tried was changing my diet and taking homeopathic supplements. These had incredible names like *Saccarromyces boulardii* and *Lactobacillus plantarum rhamnosus salivarius*. You couldn't make it up, except someone clearly has. And then there were the fertility detox diets. In one of them, food was subdivided into three groups: the green group, the blue group and the brown group. On days 1, 2, 4, 6, 9, 11, 12 and 14 you could only eat foods from the green group, and on days 3, 5, 7, 8, 10 and 13 you could eat from the green and the blue groups. Food in the brown group was forbidden at all times (no prizes for guessing that this was all the nice stuff). It was a full-time job just keeping up with the menu-planning and shopping, and then there was the cooking. I defy anyone to live this way on a long-term basis.

I think part of my problem with it all is that I've never really believed in vitamins. Throughout my adult life my eating philosophy has been to have a varied diet plus a little bit of what I fancy. Admittedly, I don't always manage five fruit and vegetable portions a day. Who does? And I'm probably a little too friendly with a few carbohydrates. But overall I think I'm pretty healthy. Consequently I found the mass of homeopathic remedies that I was prescribed a little overwhelming. I saw one nutritionist who put together a protocol for me that involved taking eighteen different supplements a day. I really liked her and she looked amazing, which made her a great advert for her own advice, but I just couldn't face putting all that stuff inside me. We had a rather awkward conversation when I received her prescription and asked her if she could recommend just one or two things off the list that she thought would really make the difference. 'No,' she said firmly. 'They are all essential.' She wouldn't back down. I didn't either.

Sometimes I wonder whether the nutritionist, like my acupuncturist, knew something about my body that I didn't. Perhaps if I had followed her combination of pills and potions to the letter things would be different. But sometimes you have to go with your gut. And my gut said no.

If you are dealing with infertility and conventional medicine doesn't work for you, it's natural to want to try other options. Added to this there is a lot of anecdotal evidence to suggest that alternative therapies can help. But when I asked my consultant in Oxford what he thought, he said: 'It makes me feel like I'm in the film *Jerry Maguire*. Do you remember the sequence when Tom Cruise is banging on the table shouting, "Show Me The Money"? Well I'm Jerry Maguire, but in my case I'm shouting, "Show Me The Evidence! SHOW ME THE EVIDENCEEEEEEEEEEEEEEE!"'

So if alternative therapies make you feel better, and you think that they are working, then carry on doing whatever you're doing. My problem is that the needles and supplements never really made me feel any different. They certainly never got me pregnant. I wish I could say that they had and that I am a living, breathing piece of anecdotal evidence. But sadly I can't.

The Infertility Diaries Part XXIV

I am longing for the day when I can attend a pregnancy yoga class. I've been doing yoga on and off for nearly twenty years and it's something I've always looked forward to. I've observed that there are two types of yoga mothers to be: the earth-mother type who wears expensive-looking floaty linen; and the sporty type who wears tight-fitting lycra-layers which show off her bump. I wonder which type of yoga-mother I'm going to be. Lately it seems as if every regular class I go to is sandwiched between a class for pregnant women. I have to admit that it's crossed my mind that I could just go along and pretend.

THE SECRET CYCLE

I try my best not to go through our next cycle. I really do. There's a lot going on in our lives. I'm back at work, busy as I ever was. Added to this, my father has had to go into hospital and we are spending all our evenings and weekends there with him.

At our follow-up appointment with the clinic they strongly advise us to have another go. They still can't offer us a diagnosis but they do suggest we throw in some immune treatment next time around, just to make sure we've covered all the bases. Like all our previous clinics they seem confident that next time it will work.

I do want to give Mr T at least one more attempt at performing his miracles on me, but I also know that our time and money is running out fast. If we are going to go through it again the timing needs to be precision perfect.

I go in for a blood test and a scan on the first day of my period. All the indications are that it would be a good month to try again. It is two months since our last cycle and, having waited an age for that to start, now everything is happening in a rush.

'To be honest, I'd rather have a break,' I say to the

doctor who sees us. 'I only want to start if it looks like it's going to be a really good month.'

'Well your blood results are excellent. Oestradiol not too high. Lots of small follicles in both ovaries. It looks like it is a good month.'

'Oh,' I say.

Later that day I get a call from the clinic.

'Mr T says you're ready to go. No down-regulation this time. Straight to stimulation. Congratulations.'

'Oh,' I say again.

Why do I sound ever so slightly disappointed? Of course I don't want to miss a good month. Not with my forty-first birthday fast approaching. Perhaps – as Peter has written in every birthday card he's given me for the last few years – this really is going to be our lucky year. I have one month left. Enough time to go through another cycle and get the results before I am yet another year older, further in debt and closer to menopause.

So, this becomes the secret cycle. I tell no one. I avoid my closest friends so I don't have to lie to them. I work right through it, shooting up in the disabled loo of the theatre like a regular drug addict. I fabricate a meeting across town so I can sneak into the clinic for a four-hour intravenous blood transfusion, which is a core part of Mr T's immune therapy. And even on the morning of egg collection I am back in work and at my desk by 10 a.m., slightly drowsy from the anaesthetic. But no one notices. At least I don't think they do.

In some ways it's just like the old days. But things have also changed. This time I know I've tried it another way. Four months off. Feet in the air. It didn't make an ounce of difference – in fact it was arguably one of the least successful cycles I've ever had. I keep thinking about all the women in the world who have sustained pregnancies in the most terrible circumstances. Running a theatre isn't going to make or break it. It's either going to work or it isn't. I'm not sure whether I've actually got anything to do with it.

The day after egg collection six out of our eight eggs have fertilised. This is a good result in our fertilisation rate stakes, and one more than last time. By Day 3 all six are still developing and the embryologist at the clinic says that Mr T is extremely pleased with their quality and has recommended that we wait until they reach blastocyst(!) before putting them back.

Day 5 arrives. A Saturday. Peter is working so I go to the clinic alone. Up until now he's always been with me for our embryo transfer. But in the same way that I've been pretty relaxed about everything else this cycle, I feel fine about this too. I settle down in the waiting room. Nervously excited. Within a few minutes one of the embryologists calls me through to the reception.

'Hi Jessica,' she says. 'How are you feeling?'

'OK,' I say. 'Well, a little bit anxious, I guess. How are they doing?'

'They're fine. All of them are still developing,' she says.

'But?' I say. I know there's going to be one. This is me, after all.

The embryologist looks at me kindly.

'Yes, but, none of them have reached blastocyst yet,' she says. 'So I think we're going to wait until tomorrow to make a decision on which to put back.'

'Tomorrow?' I say. 'That will be Day 6. Is that normal?'

'Well, not normal as such, but it can happen. It does happen. There's nothing to worry about.'

Here we go again. Nothing to worry about but something new to google: *blastocyst transfer on Day 6*. For every negative entry I find there's also a positive one, and, naturally, the obligatory story of a woman who had two blastocysts transferred on Day 6 and now has twins. But it's like spotting. Of course it doesn't necessarily mean the worst but it's also not a great sign. Our embryos are developing slower than they should, and, contrary to Aesop's fable, the tortoise doesn't always win the race.

On the bright side (the Price side), Peter will be home tomorrow and can come with me for the transfer.

Sunday morning. We arrive at the clinic for a long wait. Eventually the embryologist calls us downstairs.

'How are things today?' I ask tentatively.

I'm already practically convinced that none of them have survived and they have spent all this time planning their strategy about how they are going to tell me.

'They're fine,' she says. 'You've got a couple of really nice ones.'

'Really?' I say disbelievingly.

'Yes. Really.'

After another long wait three of our embryos are transferred. The other three are deemed not high enough quality for freezing. When we finally emerge from the clinic it's long past lunch. We're starving and the five of us (me, Peter and our three embryos) head to Soho for a burger. I've already worked out long ago that I'm going to be a junk-food-in-moderation mother. Might as well start as I mean to go on.

So here we are yet again. My ninth two-week wait. A couple of days in and I have a few tiny spots of dark brown blood. My heart sinks as I return to the Internet for what must be the millionth time to search 'spotting' and 'implantation bleeding'. Even as I'm doing it, I'm thinking: *what the hell is there that I don't already know about this subject?* But I find a new site which says that spotting a few days after transfer is much more likely to be implantation bleeding (a good sign), and spotting near to your pregnancy test date is much more likely to be the onset of your period (a bad sign). Previously I've always started spotting just a few days before I was due to test, so I decide to tell myself that it must be implantation bleeding. After a day it goes away, adding further fuel to my theory.

(OT)D-day draws closer. I buy a First Response pregnancy test. It's burning a hole in my bag as I oscillate hourly about if and when do it. Eventually I decide to do it the day before my official test day, before Peter gets home from work. Maybe this is selfish. If it's positive, I'm taking away the shared joy of seeing a double pink line. But if it's negative all I have to manage, at least for a while, is my own disappointment.

It's negative.

What did I expect?

Come on. What did you expect?

The Infertility Diaries Part XXV

My dad will be ninety-two next month. He had me in his early fifties and I spent all my childhood thinking he would die because he was so much older than all my friends' dads. But he didn't. He was blessed with good genes and was active until his late eighties, when he started to have a series of strokes. For the last few years he's been in and out of hospital, where he also contracted MRSA. I have to admit that I'm guilty of googling 'MRSA and infertility', to check whether there is any known link and I've gone and caught it. (As far as I can see there isn't.) I should add this to the list of other insane Internet searches I have done, including, 'Am I pregnant if my pee smells weird?' and 'Can too many crisps make you infertile?' Google: my doctor and my devil.

MONEY

I sat down last week and did the maths. I worked out that over the last seven years we've spent over £50,000 on IVF and fertility treatments. Fifty thousand pounds and nothing to show for it – except perhaps the ability to appear on *Mastermind* with IVF as my specialist subject.

Looking back, I don't know how we've managed

it. We have remortgaged our house (twice); taken out bank loans; borrowed money from our family (which they and we know we'll probably never be able to pay back); and maxed out the credit card. Whatever happens in the end, we will be paying back what we owe for many years to come.

I tried to arrange a balance transfer on my credit card to try to lower my interest payments. It was refused. The man at the end of the phone politely explained that he couldn't tell me why but that I could check my credit score online. It hasn't quite gone into minus figures, but I wouldn't give me any more credit either.

I know our financial situation is bad and real, but when you're going through IVF it does start to feel as if you're spending Monopoly money. You don't usually pay for the process in one lump sum, as the costs vary depending on how many drugs you need, the type of treatment you have and what day your embryos go back. Each time you go into the clinic you hand over your card for something or other. After a while you don't think about the cost, beyond perhaps feeling you've got a bargain when it's a few hundred rather than a few thousand. One day I got talking to a fellow patient. She said that she'd stopped asking the amount and, as long as they deliver her a baby at the end of it, they can take what they like. But, sadly, in this game of Monopoly you may never pass go.

Now – after my ninth unsuccessful round of treatment – I have to face the fact that even if I want to go through it all again it may be financially impossible. And even if someway, somehow we can raise the cash, I am starting to wonder whether it's worth increasing our debt even further – let's face it, probably for nothing. I know that sounds negative. I know Price Pritchett would probably have a thing or two to say about it. But there does come a point when you have to accept that, however hard you work at having a baby, it might not happen. And even if we can raise the money, the choice between going through it all again or going on an amazing holiday we'll remember for the rest of our lives is starting to feel like a tough decision. It's like *Deal or No Deal*. Do you take the Banker's offer, which is in your control, or go for the box, which isn't at all?

I take my dilemma to the monthly meeting I now have with my fellow Hoffman participants. I ask the group whether they think it is time for me to stop and get on with the rest of my life. Of course no one can give me the answer, but towards the end of our discussion someone asks what I'd do if money wasn't an issue. I surprise myself by knowing the reply instantly. There is no question in my mind that physically I can put my body through another round. There is no question in my mind that emotionally I can face it, whatever the outcome. The only thing stopping me is the money. But if money were no object, of course I'd go through it again. And again. And again. And again. Until there's no more hope.

Then I remember what my friend Ella said: it's all about the number forty-three. I've just turned forty-one. Based on most fertility statistics, I've got two years left (give or take) to have my own biological baby. At forty-three the chances of IVF being successful drop to less than 3 per cent. If it's only the money that's stopping me, then we have to do whatever we can to find it. We must keep on trying. It's too late to give up now.

The Infertility Diaries Part XXVI

I was at a talk today by a leading academic. He was speaking about the difference between things that are complicated and things that are complex. Cars and computers are complicated. It's difficult to understand how they work, but if you put in the time and effort you'll get there in the end. Things that are complex are much more difficult to fathom. There are so many subjective variables that it may be impossible to ever really know the answer. He was talking about cultural theory but it made me think about my infertility. Am I

complicated or complex? Will it ever be possible to know
the reason why?

NATURAL SELECTION

After two tries with Taranissi it's time to move on. That's not to say I wouldn't recommend him to others. But he hasn't been able to work his miracles on me. Nobody has.

We still don't have any answers. But I can tell that, despite there being no technical reason we can't get pregnant and are continuing to create beautiful embryos in the laboratory, even the doctors at Mr Taranissi's clinic – allegedly the most successful fertility clinic in the country – are starting to doubt that it's ever going to work. Perversely, perhaps, this makes me even more determined.

When I get home from work each night I go to Google for inspiration and solace. One evening I stumble on an article about a clinic which practises 'mild' and 'natural' IVF. This is basically IVF with few or no drugs. The article says that although this means you produce fewer follicles and fewer eggs, which in theory reduces the statistical chance of success, it's better for your body and improves the quality of your embryos. Whilst I've been happily pumping my body with fertility drugs for years now without giving a second thought to the long-term consequences, I am immediately struck by the quality argument. Given my advancing age, maybe our last hope is to try and harvest the best egg I can and set it up on a date with Peter's sperm.

The next day I ring the clinic and make an appointment.

I hand over my lever arch file of past notes to the director of the clinic. She's the first female fertility doctor we've seen. She's also a professor, which I guess means she must be clever.

'The results of all Peter's sperm samples seem normal,' she says, leafing through our file. 'Can I ask why you've always had ICSI?'

'Well, years ago now, we did a twenty-four-hour sperm survival test,' Peter says. 'The results indicated that my sperm didn't survive very long. Our clinic at the time recommended ICSI rather than conventional IVF, and since then every clinic we've been to has just followed suit.'

'That test has been all but discredited these days,' she says. 'At this clinic we believe in natural selection. Unless there is a clear reason for ICSI – and I don't believe there is in your case – I would recommend standard IVF in order to let the best sperm choose themselves.'

'So do you have any idea what our problem might be?' I ask her.

'It's difficult to tell. The biochemical pregnancies and miscarriage suggest there might be implantation problems. And your age now will certainly be a factor, but it wouldn't have been when you started. Maybe over the years you've had too much intervention.'

'Too much intervention? What do you mean?' I say.

'I believe that many couples are given high dosages of drugs and procedures like ICSI before it's needed. My theory is that you should start by trying as naturally as possible, using no or low levels of drugs, and work your way up from there. Not the other way around.'

She is equally definitive about Mr T's immune therapy – 'unproven and unlicensed' – and about alternative treatments like acupuncture and supplements: 'unproven and unnecessary'.

'In the first instance my recommendation would be that you undertake a cycle of mild IVF,' she says. 'This means that we will give you some stimulation drugs, but far less than you've been used to having.'

'What will that do?'

'It will induce more than one follicle, but, Jessica, you'll need to stop any obsessions you have about egg numbers,' she says pointedly. 'With natural and mild IVF we are only trying to produce a small number of eggs. We're interested in *quality* not *quantity*.'

It is as if she had read my mind, but I have to admit that the thought of it is quite liberating. After all, we only need one plus one (or, if we're double lucky, two plus two).

We decide to give the clinic a go. An added benefit is that mild IVF is cheaper than conventional IVF (on account of there being fewer drugs), and considerably cheaper than a round of treatment with Mr Taranissi (on account of there being less of everything). But it is nerve-wracking. I've now grown accustomed to the daily blood tests and scans that carefully monitored my progress. This time it's just down to me and my body, which it is now blatantly clear can't be trusted.

On egg collection day the result is five. Five eggs and I'm feeling fine. It's actually only three less than I achieved the last two times with Taranissi, on half the drugs, which does make me wonder whether we've been wasting our money all these years. After the collection one of the embryologists calls us through to discuss next steps.

'Your eggs and sperm look good,' she says. 'Having said that, I think my recommendation is that you do ICSI again rather than IVF.'

'Why?' I say confused. 'We were told that if Peter's

sperm looked fine you would do conventional IVF.'

I am surprised and a bit disappointed at the sudden change of tack.

'That's true,' she says. 'We would usually, but I'm just going on your history. At least with ICSI you know you've got a record of successful fertilisation. If we do IVF there is going to be a small danger that none of them fertilises.'

'How much of a danger?'

'Maybe about 15 per cent.'

'But at least we would learn something new,' I say.

'Yes, but you've got to think about how you would feel if you didn't have any embryos to put back. ICSI is definitely the safer bet in your case.'

She is very patient with us as we talk around and around each option. Then she suggests we go out for a walk to think about it. I can see that, when faced with a relatively small number of eggs and our past record, it might suddenly seem foolhardy to try something different. But at the same time, that's what everyone else has done and it never got me pregnant. The fresh air emboldens me. If nobody can give me the answers to why we're not getting pregnant then maybe it's time to start looking for them myself.

'I think we should risk it,' I say to Peter.

'Go against the embryologist's recommendation?'

'Coming here was about doing things differently. If none of them fertilises then at least we'll definitely know that my eggs and your sperm don't like each other. It will give us more information.'

'But how are you going to handle it if that happens?'

'My instinct is already telling me that none of them will fertilise and this round will have been for nothing…but we'll have learned something.'

We go back to the clinic and tell the embryologist. Then I all but put it out of my mind, convinced that this round of IVF is over. It feels hard, but I'm also dealing with the fact that my dad has just been taken into hospital again and is very ill. At least I won't have to cope with that alongside another two-week wait.

The next morning the phone rings at 8.20 while I'm in the bath. It's the embryologist.

'Good morning, Jessica.' She sounds a bit excited. 'Do you want to know how many embryos you have today?'

'Go on, tell me.'

'Five! All five eggs have fertilised.'

'Really?' I say incredulously.

'Really. 100 per cent success.'

'Oh my god. That's amazing. AMAZING.'

Peter rushes in from the kitchen and punches the air.

'I have to admit I was worried,' she says. 'It was the first thing I looked at when I came in this morning.'

'It's incredible. INCREDIBLE,' I say.

'It is. And just think, all those years of ICSI and you never needed it.'

I'm staggered and delighted in equal measure. In seven years it's the best fertilisation rate we have ever had.

'I am so delighted for you, Jessica,' the embryologist says. 'I will be waiting and watching for the result of your pregnancy test.'

I put down the phone. *Optimism may be good, Mr Price Pritchett, but let me tell you: there's nothing quite like pessimism when it's proved wrong.* Right now I feel like the luckiest person alive.

Peter looks at me.

'I love you,' he says. 'You made a massive decision yesterday. I love you for your bravery.'

Two days later, three of our five embryos are put back. Two grade ones, one grade two. On the dreaded Day 13 of the two-week wait I start spotting. I take a First Response pregnancy test. It's negative.

Later that day my dad dies.

Life gives and it takes away. Today it took away a lot and gave me nothing back in return. Sometimes there isn't any justice in the world.

The Infertility Diaries Part XXVII

I don't want to hear any more stories about someone's friend of a friend who tried to have a baby for years and then suddenly fell pregnant when they stopped trying. Who are these people? I don't believe that you ever stop trying.

THE OTHER OPTIONS

So when is the right time to think about the other options? Egg donation? Sperm donation? Surrogacy? Adoption? Looking back over seven fruitless years, I just wish that we had done it earlier. Now it feels as if this journey has to result in our own biological baby or nothing at all, and that's largely because I haven't got the energy to start all over again on something new.

I must know practically everything there is to know about IVF using our own eggs and sperm. But I know practically nothing about what's involved in adoption, except that it can take years and often involves intrusive interrogation by well-meaning social workers. I do understand that this is an important part of the process, but at the same time

I don't know if I would be able to hide my fear that I sometimes feel our infertility means we don't deserve to be parents and that it's nature's way of telling us that we won't make very good ones.

As for egg and sperm donation, I've always felt it was something I wouldn't consider and no one ever suggested it to us until I turned forty. But I've recently seen two great documentary films about donor conception. The first – *Donor Unknown* – was about an American guy who spent his twenties in producing rooms, ejaculating for money. At the latest count his sperm has fathered at least twelve children and the film followed their quest to find him. He's now a hippy living in a camper van on California's Venice Beach with four dogs and a pet pigeon.

The second documentary – *Donor Mum: The Children I've Never Met* – was about a woman who conceived her son through donor sperm and wanted to give something back, so she anonymously donated two of her eggs at the same time. They were given to a woman who had been involved in a plane crash in which her own two children had died and who had sustained such severe injuries herself that she was no longer able to conceive. It was the most heart-warming story, above all for the generosity and humility of the woman who had donated her eggs, and the gratitude and joy of the woman who had received them.

But despite these extraordinary and wonderful stories I still can't imagine carrying and giving birth to a child that is genetically unknown to me, especially when there are so many children around the world who have already been born and need new parents.

And then there's surrogacy. I don't even properly understand when this becomes an option. I presume it's when a woman can't carry a child herself. Surely our healthy eggs and sperm and my inhospitable womb would make us a potential candidate, yet, again, no one has ever suggested it to us.

The problem is it's difficult to navigate the other options, especially when you're diagnosed with unexplained infertility. You just keep hoping that natural or assisted conception is eventually going to work. Of all the clinics we've been to, not one of them has actively helped us to explore all the options or even contacted us six months on to find out how we are. I sometimes wonder whether all the doctors we've seen over the years ever remember us and wonder what happened. Or are we just a failed statistic that brought their year-end success rates down and then, thankfully, disappeared?

At the risk of sounding evangelical, what the world needs is a place where infertile couples can go to talk through all the options early on, with someone who is knowledgeable and understanding, who can listen to their story from all sides and explain all the possibilities. If this had been readily available to us we might have made different choices. Maybe we would have a family now – even if it wasn't biologically our own. Maybe we would have lived our life of infertility in a different way.

The Infertility Diaries Part XXVIII

The thing is we're all just specks. Specks in an infinite universe. In a hundred years' time it won't matter who had a baby and who didn't. It doesn't now. It only matters to me because in my world I am enormous. So I am trying to put things in perspective and it helps to think of myself as a speck. The important thing is to make the most of the short time I have here: to relish all the options that are possible.

601 DAYS

My dad's funeral was a perfect day. I know that sounds wrong but it's true. I read a poem; Peter did the eulogy; Frank Sinatra sang *Moon River*. I think when someone dies at ninety-two you have to make it a celebration of a long life lived. I like to imagine my dad lying there listening. He wouldn't have believed that it was him we were all there for. 'Amazing,' he would have said, in the way that he did, wide-eyed, lingering over the letters 'a' and 'z'.

My dad would have made a wonderful grandfather. He had a childlike quality and was a cross between a teddy bear and a little boy. Children loved him. And he loved them. But one of the things that made him special is that he never made me feel like I'd failed him by not giving him grandchildren. He was always proud of the things that I had done, and never thought about the things that I hadn't.

A few days after his funeral I come to a decision: it's time to stop writing. Death is a time for new beginnings, even if they're not the small pink ones I was hoping for. I always thought that as long as my story had a happy ending then I would be able to accept, maybe even appreciate, everything I've been through. I have kept writing in the hope that it would happen; that this would eventually become a book of triumph over adversity, like so many of the best life stories are. But it seems that for now, at least, it isn't.

Of course if we had considered some of the other options earlier I could perhaps have written an alternative happy ending. We might have had a little army of adopted children and I could have achieved my childhood dream of a family with seven siblings (any one of whom would legitimately have been able to win the school pumpkin).

But we never did. The fact that our infertility was and remains unexplainable; the fact that our eggs and sperm seem to make perfect embryos in the laboratory; the fact that in those early years the biochemical pregnancies, ectopic pregnancy and miscarriage seemed to be a clear indication that things would work out well in the end – these were all reasons why we continued on the fertility treatment treadmill.

One of the things I've learned during the last seven years is that there is still so much we don't know about infertility. IVF has become a ubiquitous treatment and it is undoubtedly one of the phenomenal medical success stories of the twentieth century. Since the first IVF baby, Louise Brown, was born in 1978 it is estimated that over four million babies have now been conceived through the treatment. It fills me with wonder and gratitude for Dr Robert Edwards, who pioneered the process that was initially so controversial he had to use his own sperm in his experiments. But at the same time I can't help thinking about what the next thirty years will bring. As we identify the real causes of what is now described as unexplained infertility we might also learn that IVF isn't always the solution. For many women of my age, who are struggling with infertility, it's sad to think that lots of new discoveries will be made during our lifetime but it will be far too late for us to benefit from them.

Yet, whatever mysterious thing is going on that has made it difficult for Peter and me to conceive and carry a baby to term, our ages are now undoubtedly coming into the equation. Many of the women I know who are a generation younger than me are starting to get pregnant. They are all in their early thirties and discovering, for the first time, the world of the ovulation predictor kit and sex-to-schedule. I can't help but feel that we've gone and missed our baby-boat.

Another cruel irony of this situation (if another were needed) is that, because I don't have children myself, none of this generation of younger women thinks I have any advice to give on the subject of trying to conceive. The truth is, I probably know more about trying to have a baby than most people – even those with pramfuls of them. So, just for the record, and especially for the women who are starting to experience the symptoms of infertility – the silent epidemic of our modern world – here are some of the things I know:

- Choose your clinic carefully. As consumers of the infertility industry we are still far too powerless in the face of the doctors who hold our happiness in their hands. Success rates are important but so are other things. For me, at the beginning, I needed a smaller clinic that allowed us to be involved in every aspect of our treatment. Latterly, after years of failure, I was prepared to forfeit involvement for a busier clinic that provided intensive monitoring. My dream would be to find a clinic that provided both, but as far as I know it doesn't exist yet. However, if as customers we start to demand better environments and a more individualised approach to our treatment, it will eventually happen, and with it I'm sure results will improve.

- If you are diagnosed with unexplained infertility I would certainly recommend trying natural IVF before you enter the world of high levels of drugs and intervention. Natural selection does make sense – after all, that is how it's meant to work normally. So don't let a doctor make any assumptions about what you need until you're certain you really need it.

- If at all possible, take some time off and dedicate yourself to your treatment. There's an argument that says it's not necessary, maybe that it even puts too much pressure on the process (and I do acknowledge that it didn't work for me). But remember that this is one of the most important and (if you're doing it privately) one of the most expensive things you'll ever do. You've got to give it your best shot. That means eating and drinking well; doing whatever helps you to relax; getting a regular eight hours a night. It's just so hard to do all these things when you're also juggling a stressful full-time job. So don't, at least for a while. Even if it's just so you don't have any regrets later.

- Although it's not something that is yet fully understood or acknowledged by the medical profession, I have no doubt that you need to treat the mind as well as the body. So get some help – and not just the counselling session that your clinic may or may not offer (and in my experience is unlikely to encourage actively). Infertility has a huge effect on your mental health and on your relationship. It can bring you together. It can push you apart. Either way, I can't recommend highly enough the benefits of having an independent, unbiased, non-judgemental witness to help you process what you're going through.

- And finally, talk about it. To yourself; to friends and family; to other people going through infertility. It took me such a long time to do this. I didn't want anyone to feel sorry for me. I didn't want to be anyone's source of schadenfreude. But over time the truth seeped out. Sometimes via circumstances I had no control over, sometimes when I made a conscious decision to be open. Looking back, I believe that the years of hiding the truth had a profound psychological and possibly physiological effect on my ability to conceive. The more we open up, the easier it is for ourselves and others. Of course no one yet knows what effects secrecy and shame have on fertility, but I bet they don't help. That's not to say you have to start wearing the infertility badge with pride. But put it on. Recognise it is part of who you are. It will make it easier for others to do the same.

So, having made the decision to end it – this story, that is – I go to a café after work one evening, open my laptop and put fingers to keys.

Nothing comes.

For the first time in years, I realise there is no plan formulating in my mind about what to do next. Should we try again? Should we give up? Or has the moment finally come to explore all the alternative possibilities – including a life without children? And maybe I don't want a baby anyway? Do I really want to have my sleeping patterns disrupted; become acquainted with the perils of childcare; give up my evenings and weekends to swimming lessons and games on Wii? Childlessness is actually starting to feel comfortable.

In a few weeks' time Peter and I have our follow-up appointment at the clinic. Will our 100 per cent fertilisation success using conventional IVF rather than ICSI give us anything new to go on? Or will we continue to be a complex case that no one seems fully able to understand or explain? Time is ticking and I know that someone soon is going to say that it's up; that sadly my age and medical science ultimately failed to coalesce. There are only 601 days to go. Six hundred and one days until I reach that all-important number forty-three.

I close my laptop and head home for supper. Peter's cooking what we call a 'Peter Special' from his repertoire of six dishes. We open a bottle of wine and toast my dad and the future. Later that night, as I get into bed, I look at the little pile of list books that is always on the table beside my pillow. I pick up the one with all the countries I've ever visited and then go and get our atlas from the bookshelf in the hall. I open it and start to trace my fingers across the coloured continents. I remember how as a teenager I told my careers adviser that I wanted to run a theatre or become an expedition leader. How motherhood never figured.

Sometimes the things you take for granted in life

end up being the things you want the most and have least control over. But if I haven't had a baby by the time I'm forty-three, then perhaps I can travel the world instead. By my latest count I've visited thirty countries, which leaves about another 170 to go. Being able to say I've travelled to every country in the world – now *that* would be something.

The Infertility Diaries Part XXIX

Infertility has made me into a gambler. I have started to buy lottery scratch cards in the hope of winning £100,000 to feed my IVF habit or, alternatively, buy a round-the-world-ticket when I'm forty-three. Today I won £1. At least it's a start.

BLESSINGS

I've recently started a new list book. I call it my Blessings Book. It's become an important reminder for me that, despite my infertility, there's still something to bless in every day. Sometimes a day seems so perfect that I have to include every detail. Other days it might be just a great cup of coffee, the colour of spring blossom, or the kindness of a stranger.

Looking back, there are many reasons to bless my infertility. If I had got pregnant when we first started trying I'm not sure I could have carried on doing the job I do now. Peter and I have visited some incredible places that we probably would have never been able to go to if we had children. And I now know so much more about myself than I did before I started this journey. If I'm given the chance, I'm sure that it will make me a better mother.

In the darkest moments, my Blessings Book has become a reminder of all the things in life to be grateful for. If you desperately want a baby but can't get pregnant, it's going to be one of the really sad things in your life. But juxtapose it with everything that makes life worth living. We're not working towards a happy ending. Life is not linear. There will be good times then bad times. Bad times then good. So count your blessings wherever you find them and enjoy the journey wherever it takes you. Because life is a blessing that has been given to us by our parents. Even if we can't pass it on as parents ourselves.

The Infertility Diaries Part XXX

And…if I'm blessed with a miracle in the next 601 days, I'll be the happiest person alive. But you won't find me posting our scan photos on Facebook or rubbing my burgeoning belly in meetings. I'll always be the Infertile Mother. It's who I've become.

EPILOGUE

601 days and counting (down)

When we go to see our consultant she says that our results are unfathomable. Like us, she is astounded by our 100 per cent fertilisation success rate with conventional IVF. But she still doesn't have any answers. In fact, to our shock and surprise, her conclusion is that the time has come to give up. She says there's no scientific explanation for why we can't conceive, but there's no denying ten rounds of unsuccessful treatment either.

When she sees our crestfallen faces she softens slightly and suggests that we go for one final opinion. She recommends a doctor who has been having phenomenal results with an obscure form of mushroom therapy. I know. *Mushrooms.* Are there truly no limits to which women will go to have a baby?

This particular doctor's practice is in the picturesque village of Petersham, although it looks like it should be in the Hollywood Hills. The front door opens on to a long, white, roof-lit corridor lined with contemporary art. It's achingly cool and modern.

He reviews our history with interest – even calls over his nurse to look at the grainy picture of my abdominal ectopic, describing it as extremely rare and absolutely fascinating. I puff up with pride. He then says that he thinks the results from our past treatment are collectively significant and that he would like us to do another round of tests before coming back for a full diagnosis. He says that he's pretty sure we are creating perfect embryos, but something is happening when they get to my womb that is stopping their growth and survival. He's convinced that the reason why our ectopic embryo did so well is because it was outside my womb, where it was safe.

So we do the tests and, astonishingly, one of them throws up a result – it's an obscure immune test that we've never had before, not even with the controversial Mr T. And this new doctor, who I have decided is just a little bit magic, gives us the first ever definitive diagnosis of our case.

It goes like this.

When you have an embryo developing inside your womb, you rely on your immune system to tell you to protect it and not to fight it. Most of the fertility immune testing that is done at the moment (and remember there isn't very much of it) measures the cells that fight. Hardly any measures the cells that protect. In our case the fighting part of my immune system seems to be fine but the protecting part is atrocious.

The doctor tells us that he is convinced that the result is important and that there is no point in trying to get pregnant, either naturally or via IVF, until the problem is resolved. He even says that, starting from today, we need to discount everything that has gone before – all seven and a half years of it – because today is the first day of our new pregnancy journey.

After all this time, to be finally given an answer – whether it is true or not, curable or not – is incredible. It should feel unfair, upsetting, un-understandable, but in fact it's liberating. No more IVF. No more unexplainable disappointment. Not until we fix the problem. If we can.

The doctor then tells us that there are currently only two, scientifically unproven, ways to do this. The first is his bizarre concoction of Chinese mushrooms. The second is an even more bizarre and controversial process which involves removing Peter's or another man's white blood cells and injecting them into me. He says he's convinced that if either of these treatments works then we will get pregnant and might not even need IVF.

I've been through enough to know that it's far too risky to believe in miracles, but after years of knowing nothing it's just wonderful to think we might finally know something. And when you think about it logically, it does kind of make sense that your immune system would have an important effect on your fertility. After all, it's supposed to fight off illness and infection, and an embryo is essentially an alien cell. It figures that your body needs to be able to tell itself to protect and not to attack.

So right now we're on those mushrooms, and if that doesn't work we'll contemplate the blood transfusion. I quite like the thought of Peter's blood cells mingling with mine, making friends, and encouraging each other to protect our foetus when it comes along.

We shall see. From now on, it's all about the number forty-three. My own special 'prime number', divisible only by me. It's when my pursuit of motherhood ends and a new life begins – I just don't know yet whether it's going to be my life or someone else's.

Acknowledgements

Special thanks to my friends – Beth, Ella, Tara and Vicky – for agreeing to appear in the book and for all their support over many years. Thank you also to all the other friends, family and colleagues who make anonymous appearances. I am also extremely grateful to Price Pritchett for allowing me to reproduce excerpts from his book Hard Optimism (these are used with full permission of Pritchett, LP and all rights are reserved).

For their brilliant professional advice, thanks to Diana Beaumont, Polly Courtney, Charlotte Macpherson, Helen McCusker, Richard Spence, Emily Sweet, Justine Taylor and the whole team at Troubador Publishing.

And finally to Peter. For being my first reader and supporting me to tell our story in my words.